THE MEDICAL LIBRARY ASSOCIATION GUIDE TO PROVIDING CONSUMER AND PATIENT HEALTH INFORMATION

Medical Library Association Books

The Medical Library Association (MLA) features books that showcase the expertise of health sciences librarians for other librarians and professionals.

MLA Books are excellent resources for librarians in hospitals, medical research practice, and other settings. These volumes will provide health care professionals and patients with accurate information that can improve outcomes and save lives.

Each book in the series has been overseen editorially since conception by the Medical Library Association Books Panel, composed of MLA members with expertise spanning the breadth of health sciences librarianship.

Medical Library Association Books Panel

Carol Ann Attwood, AHIP, chair
Barbara Gushrowski, chair designate
Gail Y. Hendler
Megan Curran Rosenbloom
Tracy Shields
Kristen L. Young, AHIP
Lauren M. Young, AHIP
Gabriel R. Rios, board liaison

About the Medical Library Association

Founded in 1898, MLA is a 501(c)(3) nonprofit, educational organization of 4,000 individual and institutional members in the health sciences information field that provides lifelong educational opportunities, supports a knowledge-base of health information research, and works with a global network of partners to promote the importance of quality information for improved health to the health care community and the public.

Books in Series

The Medical Library Association Guide to Providing Consumer and Patient Health Information edited by Michele Spatz
Health Sciences Librarianship edited by M. Sandra Wood

THE MEDICAL LIBRARY ASSOCIATION GUIDE TO PROVIDING CONSUMER AND PATIENT HEALTH INFORMATION

Edited by Michele Spatz

ROWMAN & LITTLEFIELD
Lanham • Boulder • New York • Toronto • Plymouth, UK

Published in cooperation with the Medical Library Association

Published by Rowman & Littlefield
4501 Forbes Boulevard, Suite 200, Lanham, Maryland 20706
www.rowman.com

10 Thornbury Road, Plymouth PL6 7PP, United Kingdom

Copyright © 2014 by Medical Library Association

British Library Cataloguing in Publication Information Available

Library of Congress Cataloging-in-Publication Data

The Medical Library Association guide to providing consumer and patient health information / edited by Michele Spatz.
    p. ; cm.—(Medical Library Association books)
  Guide to providing consumer and patient health information
  Includes bibliographical references and index.
  ISBN 978-1-4422-3070-5 (cloth : alk. paper)—ISBN 978-1-4422-2570-1 (paper : alk. paper)—ISBN 978-1-4422-2571-8 (electronic)
  I. Spatz, Michele, 1954– editor of compilation. II. Medical Library Association, sponsoring body. III. Title: Guide to providing consumer and patient health information. IV. Series: Medical Library Association books.
  [DNLM: 1. Consumer Health Information. 2. Library Services. 3. Patient Education as Topic. WA 590]
  RA440.5
  362.1—dc23   2014003614

♾™ The paper used in this publication meets the minimum requirements of American National Standard for Information Sciences—Permanence of Paper for Printed Library Materials, ANSI/NISO Z39.48-1992.

Printed in the United States of America

Contents

Figures and Tables

Figures

Tables

Preface

Each day, in the course of their work, countless librarians work with healthcare consumers and patients alike, providing invaluable assistance in locating meaningful health information. For some librarians, this is par for the course. For others, it's challenging on many levels: they may be new to the field, lack confidence in their skill set, not know what key resources are available, nor understand how to conduct a reference interview. They may be uncomfortable dealing with someone whose needs are complex or who speaks a different language.

While we learn immensely by doing, a common knowledge base will help us hone our skills more quickly and build our expertise in this important area of librarianship by providing a solid foundation for a knowledgeable and compassionate practice.

Composed of thirteen chapters written by experienced consumer health librarians, this book is designed for library and information science graduate students as well as librarians new to health and medical librarianship, regardless of library setting. It is comprehensive in scope, covering all aspects of consumer and patient health and medical information from their humble, grassroots beginnings to the ever-evolving applications of new technology and social media. In between, the mundane aspects of health and medical librarianship, such as needs assessment, costs, budgeting and funding, and staffing are discussed. Adding richness to this discussion are the coverage of more sensitive topics such as patient-friendly technology, ethical issues in providing consumer and patient health information, meeting the needs of diverse populations, and responding to individuals from various cultural backgrounds. No comprehensive picture of consumer and patient health librarianship would be complete without addressing the critical importance of marketing and strategic partnerships; such discussions round out this volume.

Patients today must be knowledgeable enough to participate in their health and well-being. Shorter hospital stays, changing reimbursement patterns, and the gradual shift towards focusing on proactively maintaining health and managing disease require patients to be informed *and* actively engaged. Education, information, and understanding are important components of actively engaged patients. Correspondingly, in today's e-world, there is a glut of information resources available through the Internet—from YouTube videos to Googling to blogs and Twitter feeds. What is lacking in these information-rich times is the relevance of meaning and context for those who ask, "Does this health and medical information apply to me and my unique clinical picture?" or "How do I use this information?" As knowledge navigators, information technology wizards, and content experts, librarians offer focused responses to individuals' specific and highly personal health and medical information queries. In a new healthcare world order of optimizing health and minimizing hospitalizations, such a service is invaluable.

Sadly, there still exists in our highly networked and technological age an information gap for those who struggle in obtaining meaningful health or medical information. These individuals may be foreign-born, non-English speaking, poor, rural, aged, or semi-literate. Whatever their status, librarians must have the wherewithal to find germane resources and also help create responsive mechanisms to bridge that health information gap for vulnerable citizens.

When all is said and done, librarians form relationships with others. All of our savvy tech skills and ability to organize and assimilate complex information are for naught if we are not connected with others—either virtually or face-to-face. Humanity is the common currency that enriches our work. By bringing our unique skills to bear in our relationships to patients and healthcare consumers, we assist real people in acquiring information, resources, and materials with which to better understand their health, make decisions, or spark a dialogue with their healthcare provider. In service to others, we strive to achieve our profession's noble purpose.

The Medical Library Association's Policy Statement, *The Librarian's Role in the Provision of Consumer Health Information and Patient Education* (http://caphis.mlanet.org/chis/librarian.html [accessed October 23, 2012]) identifies six important responsibilities for today's consumer health librarians: collection management, knowledge and resource sharing, advocacy, access and dissemination of information, education, and research. To that end, may this book help provide a foundation, a humble beginning if you will, upon which to build an enduring approach to the practice of consumer and patient librarianship.

I'd like to commend the chapter authors for contributing their expertise to *The Medical Library Association Guide to Providing Consumer and Patient Health Information.* It is through the gracious sharing of their knowledge and experience in the field that a solid foundation and path for others to follow is laid.

Michele Spatz
Editor

Acknowledgments

I N GRATITUDE TO MY HUSBAND, Daniel Spatz, and to my contributors, who made the existence of this book possible.

1

History of Consumer and Patient Health Librarianship

Michele Spatz

IN UNDERSTANDING THE GROWTH OF consumer health information, it's important to remember that its roots are intertwined with the history of medicine itself. As recently as the late 1990s, it wasn't easy to find medical information in lay language. An article by August La Rocco in the January 1994 issue of the *Bulletin of the Medical Library Association* briefly describes how medicine, throughout history, was closed off and deemed inaccessible to the average individual. Medicine was shrouded in secrecy and, hence, information belonged to a privileged circle. Medicine men were apprenticed in their work and carefully chosen (La Rocco, 1994). The motto of the day was, "May he who knows, instruct him who knows. And him who knows not, not read this" (Siegerist, 1951, as cited by La Rocco, 1994, p. 46).

La Rocco illustrates this secrecy, describing how early prescriptions were written in Latin so the patient would not know the specifics of treatment and, accordingly, could not participate in the decision-making process (La Rocco, 1994). The complexity of medical language limited the layperson's understanding. For hundreds of years, medicine's early roots entwined men and magic to shape our early perceptions of who should have access to knowledge *so closely linked with life and death.*

In looking at medicine's historical timeline, it is only in the past century that it truly became grounded in empirical evidence and thus, a scientific discipline. Once fully grounded in science, medicine grew rapidly through revolutionary discoveries (e.g., germ theory, the importance of sterilization, and the development of antibiotics). As the body of medical knowledge grew, the discipline of medicine branched out from a general practice into specialized areas of concentration. Advancing technology, including the introduction of computers, added to medicine's pioneering accomplishments as well as its complexity. For all its achievements in the last half of the twentieth century, medicine was still a world very much closed off to the average American . . . or was it?

Parallel to the incredible medical advances over the past fifty years was the rise of empowered consumers. Their pressure has reshaped American medicine and lifted its shroud of secrecy. In modern America, an early example of the current consumer health movement can be seen in the radical decade of the 1960s, with its budding feminist movement, consciousness-raising sessions, and focus on personal health and well-being. During this time, women began to question medical practices. They wanted to be active, not passive, recipients of medical care. Women's groups met and discussed health issues and female anatomy. In response to the lack of lay health information available to women, the Boston Women's Health Collective organized and published the landmark book, *Our Bodies, Ourselves.* It was written "by women, for women" (Boston Women's Health Book Collective, 1973) and in its frank and unabashed style ushered in a new era of consumer health information.

As women became more informed and empowered during the 1970s, the United States saw dramatic shifts in obstetrics care as the nation's hospitals transformed their labor and delivery departments. Prior to consumer demand, hospital maternity units were places where women were anesthetized and delivered under sedation, while husbands paced outside the unit's doors waiting for their baby to be born. Women, in a sense, rebelled against the pendulum swing in medicine that had changed something perfectly natural—childbirth—into something which required hospitalization and separation from their loved ones. In answer to consumer dissatisfaction and pressure, hospital maternity units quickly evolved into "birthing centers" with fathers not only present, but active participants as coaches, supporters, and sometimes, umbilical cord cutters. The potential loss of the childbirth market to outside providers (e.g., midwives and home births) caused the medical establishment to respond to the public's demand to make childbirth more "natural" and family oriented.

With each success, the consumer health movement, which includes lay health information, began to grow. In 1973, the American Hospital Association published its first "Patient's Bill of Rights," which stated "the patient has the right to receive from his physician complete current information concerning his diagnosis, treatment and prognosis in language the patient can reasonably be expected to understand" (American Hospital Association, 1973). This first bill of rights was designed to make patient care more effective and was considered groundbreaking at the time. It has since been revised and renamed "The Patient Care Partnership." Written in plain language and translated into seven languages, it's meant to facilitate communication between patients and caregivers (American Hospital Association, 2003).

Other organizations followed suit by promoting patient access to information in their policy-making. In the early 1990s, the Joint Commission on the Accreditation of Healthcare Organizations (JCAHO, now known simply as the Joint Commission) added a section to its standards addressing patient and family education and access to health information. The American Association of Family Physicians noted in its 1995 Statement on Patient Education, "Providing patients with complete and current information helps create an atmosphere of trust, enhances the doctor-patient relationship and empowers patients to participate in their own health care" (American Association of Family Physicians, 1995).

Patient access to information was also an integral part of the philosophy of patient-centered care. The whole notion of patient-centered care started as a grassroots movement. One early effort began with a patient named Angelica Thieriot, who experienced a lengthy hospital stay in the mid-1970s that she found to be lacking in humanity. When she regained her health, Angelica formed a nonprofit organization called Planetree, named for the sycamore tree beneath which Hippocrates is believed to have taught his medical students in ancient Greece. Hoping to reconnect modern technologically focused medical care with its early roots of healing the whole person, Planetree's goal is to transform patients' experience of healthcare through personalizing, humanizing, and demystifying medicine. One of the organization's first steps was to open a consumer health library, a radical notion at the time (Planetree, 2013). Providing patients with access to both the technical and lay medical literature was viewed as a constructive step by Planetree's founders in demystifying healthcare for consumers, fully expecting once they were knowledgeable about their illness or condition, patients could actively participate in their healthcare conversations and decisions.

In 1996, as the twentieth century drew to a close, the Institute of Medicine empaneled a group of experts to address its long-term initiative focused on assessing and improving the nation's quality of care. In its landmark report on the state of healthcare delivery in the United States, *Crossing the Quality Chasm* (2001), it noted, "As medical science and technology have advanced at a rapid pace . . . the health care delivery system has floundered in its ability to provide consistently high-quality care to all Americans" (Institute of Medicine, 2001). The Institute of Medicine stated the key strategies necessary for building a more responsive healthcare system included:

- Giving patients the necessary information and the opportunity to exercise the degree of control they choose over healthcare decisions that affect them.
- Encouraging shared decision-making and patients' ability to access their own medical information.
- Fostering effective communication with their healthcare team by providing patients access to clinical knowledge.
- Establishing the provision of appropriate patient or consumer health information and patient participation in decision-making as critical tools for improving healthcare delivery (Institute of Medicine, 2001).

Along with healthcare quality issues facing U.S. healthcare consumers was the recognition that lifestyle choices were costing lives. In the early 1990s, McGinnis and Foege did an extensive study examining the causes of death in the United States (McGinnis and Foege, 1993). This study was repeated years later by Mokdad et al. who found "about half of all deaths that occurred in the United States in 2000 could be attributed to a limited number of largely preventable behaviors and exposures. Overall, we found relatively minor changes from 1990 to 2000 in the estimated number of deaths due to actual causes" (Mokdad, Marks, Stroup, and Gerberding, 2004). In both studies, the leading causes of death are linked to the *personal health choices people make*—tobacco use, poor eating habits, lack of physical exercise, and alcohol abuse (McGinnis and Foege, 1993; Mokdad, Marks, Stroup, and Gerberding, 2004).

Knowledge and information alone will not change behavior but they are part of an important first step in the process of self-change (Prochaska, 1994). While this is an important truth, some individuals lack the skills for self-empowerment. In its landmark report, *Health Literacy: A Prescription to End Confusion*, the Institute of Medicine states, "studies have shown that people with low health literacy understand health information less well, get less preventive care—such as screenings for cancer—and use expensive health services such as emergency department care more frequently" (Nielson-Bohlman et al., 2004). In fact, the economic burden of not meeting patients' health literacy needs costs the United States an estimated $106 billion to $238 billion annually, representing between 7 and 17 percent of all personal healthcare expenditures, according to an economic impact report led by a University of Connecticut economist (Vernon, Trujillo, Rosenbaum, and DeBuono, 2007).

About the same time as the economic impact of health literacy was making headlines, the Joint Commission released its white paper, "What Did the Doctor Say? Improving Health Literacy to Protect Patient Safety," stressing there is a "fundamental right and need for patients to receive information—

both orally and written—about their care in a way in which they can understand this information." The white paper goes on to state, "the safety of patients cannot be assured without mitigating the negative effects of low health literacy" (Joint Commission, 2007). Engaging patients in their learning and meeting their health information needs is part of the recommended strategy to reach national patient safety goals and reduce the nation's healthcare costs.

These concepts of patient engagement and empowerment as mechanisms to help address the nation's healthcare woes became a hallmark of national health policy as healthcare costs continued to tax the U.S. economy. According to a Kaiser U.S. Healthcare Cost Background Brief, "health expenditures in the United States neared $2.6 trillion in 2010, over ten times the $256 billion spent in 1980" (KaiserEdu.org, 2013). In 2010, the U.S. Congress passed the Patient Protection and Affordable Care Act (H.R. 3590, 2010) followed by the Health Care and Education Reconciliation Act of 2010 (H.R. 4872, 2010). Together, these two pieces of legislation ushered in healthcare reform in America. Designed to help consumers and also create innovative methods to reduce healthcare costs, these new laws offer healthcare benefits to previously uncovered citizens as well as protections from insurance abuse for all Americans. To reduce the burden of healthcare costs, healthcare reform measures put a greater emphasis on preventive care, effectively managing care for the chronically ill and successfully overseeing patients' transitions of care from one healthcare setting to another.

Healthcare reform has seen the advent of accountable care organizations (ACOs). The Centers for Medicare and Medicaid Services defines an ACO as "groups of doctors, hospitals, and other health care providers, who come together voluntarily to give coordinated high quality care to the Medicare patients they serve. Coordinated care helps ensure that patients, especially the chronically ill, get the right care at the right time, with the goal of avoiding unnecessary duplication of services and preventing medical errors. When an ACO succeeds in both delivering high-quality care and spending health care dollars more wisely, it will share in the savings it achieves for the Medicare program" (Centers for Medicare and Medicaid Services, 2013). To participate in the Shared Savings Program, the ACO must define, establish, implement, and periodically update processes to promote patient engagement, including:

- Providing understandable communication of clinical knowledge/evidence-based medicine to patients.
- Participating in shared decision-making that takes into account patients' needs, preferences, values, and priorities.
- Using decision-support tools and shared decision-making as a method for engaging patients.

Healthcare reform also fueled development of the patient-centered medical home where patient services are team based, coordinated, accessible, and patient centered. A crucial aspect of the patient-centered medical home is "a partnership among practitioners, patients, and their families [which] ensures that decisions respect patients' wants, needs, and preferences, and that patients have the education and support they need to make decisions and participate in their own care" (Patient-Centered Primary Care Collaborative, 2013).

Today, patient-centered care is at the forefront of the nation's conversation on healthcare delivery as an important approach to meeting national health goals. Donald Berwick, former administrator of the Centers for Medicare and Medicaid Services, wrote, "'Patient-centeredness' is a dimension of health care quality in its own right, not just because of its connection with other desired aims, like safety and effectiveness. Its proper incorporation into new health care designs will involve some radical, unfamiliar, and disruptive shifts in control and power, out of the hands of those who give care and into the hands of those who receive it. Such a consumerist view of the quality of care, itself, has important differences from the more classical, professionally dominated definitions of 'quality'" (Berwick, 2009, p. w555).

Of note, of course, is that as healthcare consumerism grew, librarians responded by creating innovative programs and services. Early efforts included public, hospital, or health sciences library partnerships such as the Consumer Health Information Program and Services/Salud y Bienestar in Los Angeles, California; the Community Health Information Network in Cambridge, Massachusetts; the InfoHealth Project in Cleveland, Ohio; and the collaboration of the New York Onondaga County Public Library and Consumer Health Information Consortium in Syracuse, New York (Yi, 2012).

In 1984, the Medical Library Association established its Consumer and Patient Health Information Section to provide a "forum for health sciences librarians in the area of consumer and patient health information by encouraging the formation of guidelines for the provision of consumer and patient health information, promoting the education of health sciences librarians in the provision of such information, and providing a program on consumer and patient health information at the association's annual meeting" (Medical Library Association, 2013).

The advent and evolution of the Internet during the 1990s accelerated consumers' ability to access health information and also librarians' role in assisting them. In 1996, the Consumer and Patient Health Information Section/Medical Library Association issued its first policy statement on "The Librarian's Role in the Provision of Consumer Health Information and Patient Education" (Consumer and Patient Health Information Section/Medical Library Association, 1996) to define consumer health information, patient education, and potential roles for librarians in providing these services. The defined roles encompassed collection management, knowledge and resource sharing, advocacy, access and dissemination of information, education, and research. About this time, the National Library of Medicine's strategic long-range plan made a historic shift by including as a priority the provision of health information to the general public. In the fall of 1998, the National Library of Medicine launched MedlinePlus, its groundbreaking, comprehensive medical and health information website for the public (National Library of Medicine, 2011).

To fulfill its mission of educating librarians to effectively deliver consumer health information services, the Medical Library Association began its Consumer Health Information Specialization program in 2003. The goals of the Consumer Health Information Specialization program are to equip librarians to improve health information services for consumers and keep them up to date by providing continuing education courses on new consumer health information trends and technology (Medical Library Association, 2012).

While healthcare reform takes root and ushers in a new era of patient-centered care, engagement, and empowerment, consumers today are asked to take more ownership of their health for two reasons: to reduce the burden of healthcare costs to society and to ease human suffering. Knowledge, information, and self-awareness are crucial elements of personal health ownership and self-care. In light of these mandates, consumers face mounting pressures in today's healthcare marketplace. They are expected to be informed participants in their care, discerning healthcare shoppers, *and* able to responsibly and consciously modify their lifestyle to maintain their personal health and quality of life. The demand for health information for consumers and patients has never been greater, and librarians are integral to helping them find quality resources that speak to their individual needs. Librarians provide professional navigation of evidence-based knowledge resources and help users make sense of the glut of information available. Librarians also assist consumers in their discovery of health information and the evaluation of its quality by teaching them essential skills to use technology and cultivating the discernment needed to wisely assess resources.

Libraries continue to be perceived as trustworthy places of unbiased, quality information, and as such remain a natural oasis for reliable consumer health information. Mary Jo Deering stated years ago, "as information organizers and managers, libraries bring helpful structure to the disparate mass of health information." She went on to say, "as information retrieval specialists, librarians couple an ability to clarify the patron's real health question (*as opposed to the question initially posed*) with search mapping skills to help locate the most useful information" (Deering, 1996, p. 207). Her words still ring true today for librarians as health information knowledge navigators both within and beyond the confines of the library.

Access to consumer and patient health information has grown from a simple grassroots movement to an integral part of personal health management, strategically important in meeting the Affordable Care Act's National Quality Strategy of better care, healthy people/healthy communities, and affordable care. Among its six priorities are:

- Making care safer by reducing harm caused in the delivery of care.
- Ensuring that each person and family are engaged as partners in care.
- Promoting effective communication and coordination of care.
- Promoting the most effective prevention and treatment practices for the leading causes of mortality, starting with cardiovascular disease.
- Working with communities to promote wide use of best practices to enable healthy living.
- Making quality care more affordable for individuals, families, employers, and governments by developing and spreading new healthcare delivery models (Agency for Healthcare Research and Quality, 2013).

As the pages of this book will attest, there is much librarians can and are doing to address these national health priorities by helping consumers overcome the obstacles of health literacy, cultural and language barriers, and technology in their quest to find meaningful health information. Librarians have long been community partners with their mission of providing health information. Today they are expanding upon this traditional role through health education programming, support group meeting space, and health information services including mobile technology and point-of-service programs at community locations. Always mission driven and service oriented, librarians will continue to meet consumers' and patients' evolving health and medical information needs in creative and significant ways.

References

Agency for Healthcare Research and Quality. 2013. "National Quality Strategy: Overview PowerPoint. AHRQ Working for Quality Toolkit." August 2013. http://www.ahrq.gov/workingforquality/toolkit.htm. Accessed September 8, 2013.

American Association of Family Physicians Core Educational Guideline. 1995. "Patient Education Recommended Core Educational Guidelines for Family Practice Residents." *American Family Physician*, 51(8):2012–23.

American Hospital Association. 1973. "A Patient's Bill of Rights." http://www.patienttalk.info/AHA-Patient_Bill_of_Rights.htm. Accessed September 2, 2013.

American Hospital Association. 2003. "The Patient Care Partnership. Understanding Expectations, Rights and Responsibilities." http://www.aha.org/advocacy-issues/communicatingpts/pt-care-partnership.shtml. Accessed September 5, 2013.

Berwick, DM. 2009. "What 'Patient-Centered' Should Mean: Confessions of an Extremist." *Health Affairs*, 28(4):w555–w565. http://content.healthaffairs.org/content/28/4/w555.full.html. Accessed September 8, 2013.

Boston Women's Health Book Collective. 1973. *Our Bodies, Ourselves*. New York: Simon & Schuster.

Consumer and Patient Health Information Section/Medical Library Association. 1996. "The Librarian's Role in the Provision of Consumer Health Information and Patient Education." *Bulletin of the Medical Library Association*, 84(2):238–39.

Centers for Medicare and Medicaid Services. 2013. "Accountable Care Organizations (ACOs): General Information." http://innovation.cms.gov/initiatives/aco/. Accessed September 7, 2013.

Deering, MJ. 1996. "Introduction: Partnerships for Networked Health Information for the Public." *Bulletin of the Medical Library Association*, 82(2): 206–7.

H.R. 3590. 2010. "The Patient Protection and Affordable Care Act." One Hundred Eleventh Congress of the United States of America. http://www.gpo.gov/fdsys/pkg/BILLS-111hr3590enr/pdf/BILLS-111hr3590enr.pdf. Accessed September 7, 2013.

H.R. 4872. 2010. "Health Care and Education Reconciliation Act of 2010." http://www.gpo.gov/fdsys/pkg/BILLS-111hr4872rh/pdf/BILLS-111hr4872rh.pdf. Accessed September 7, 2013.

Institute of Medicine. 2001. *Crossing the Quality Chasm: A New Health System for the 21st Century*. Committee on Quality Health Care in America, Institute of Medicine. Washington, DC: National Academies Press. http://www.nap.edu/catalog/10027.html. Accessed September 7, 2013.

Joint Commission. 2007. "What Did the Doctor Say? Improving Health Literacy to Protect Patient Safety." http://www.jointcommission.org/What_Did_the_Doctor_Say/. Accessed September 7, 2013.

KaiserEdu.org. 2013. "U.S. Healthcare Costs Background Brief." http://www.kaiseredu.org/issue-modules/us-health-care-costs/background-brief.aspx. Accessed September 7, 2013.

La Rocco, A. 1994. "The Role of the Medical School-Based Consumer Health Information Service." *Bulletin of the Medical Library Association*, 82(1):46–51.

McGinnis, JM, and Foege, WH. 1993. "Actual Causes of Death in the United States." *JAMA*, 270:2207–12.

Medical Library Association. 2012. "History of the Association: MLA Milestones: 2003." http://www.mlahq.org/about/history/milestones.html. Accessed September 7, 2013.

Medical Library Association. 2013. "Consumer and Patient Health Information Section. Description." http://www.mlanet.org/sections/secinfo1.html#consumer. Accessed September 8, 2013.

Mokdad, AH, Marks, JS, Stroup, DF, and Gerberding, JL. 2004. "Actual Causes of Death in the United States, 2000." *JAMA*, 291(10):1238–45.

National Library of Medicine. 2011. "175 Years. Our Milestones. United States National Library of Medicine 1836–2011." U.S. National Library of Medicine, National Institutes of Health. http://apps.nlm.nih.gov/175/milestones.cfm. Accessed September 7, 2013.

Nielsen-Bohlman, L, et al., eds. 2004. *Health Literacy: A Prescription to End Confusion.* Committee on Health Literacy, Institute of Medicine. Washington, DC: National Academies Press. http://www.nap.edu/catalog/10883.html. Accessed September 7, 2013.

Patient-Centered Primary Care Collaborative. 2013. "Defining the Medical Home." http://www.pcpcc.org/about/medical-home. Accessed September 7, 2013.

Planetree. 2013. "Planetree Pioneers: Angelica Thieriot." http://planetree.org/?page_id=68. Accessed September 8, 2013.

Prochaska, JO. 1994. *Changing for Good.* New York: Avon.

Siegerist, HE. 1951. *A History of Medicine.* New York: Oxford University Press.

Vernon, J, Trujillo, A, Rosenbaum, S, and DeBuono, B. 2007. "Low Health Literacy: Implications for National Health Policy." http://www.pfizerhealthliteracy.com/physicians-providers/LowHealthLiteracy.aspx. Accessed September 7, 2013.

Yi, YJ. 2012. "Consumer Health Information Behavior in Public Libraries: A Mixed Methods Study." *Electronic Theses, Treatises and Dissertations.* Paper 5290. http://diginole.lib.fsu.edu/cgi/viewcontent.cgi?article=6806&context=etd. Accessed September 8, 2013.

2

Where to Start? Needs Assessment

Nicole Dettmar

Introduction

IT IS EXCITING, AND MAY SOMETIMES SEEM overwhelming, to identify library patrons' consumer health information needs and then develop the appropriate health information collections and outreach services to meet these needs. Often, patrons already know—or at least, think they know—precisely what resources they want in terms of specific books, magazines, and online resources, as they are "constantly receiving information from the media, websites, friends and family as well as healthcare providers" (Dey, 2004, p. 121). Librarians are well positioned to help patrons find reliable, accurate, and accessible consumer health information. But first, it's essential for librarians to invest sufficient time and resources in learning more about their community through a comprehensive needs assessment.

Many librarians may feel apprehensive about needs assessment, believing this requires a complicated survey, hours of staff time, and no clear way of interpreting the results. This assumption is unfounded. A definition of needs assessment within the context of establishing benchmarks for libraries offers a framework and assurance: *a systematic process for determining discrepancies between optimal and actual performance of a service by reviewing the service needs of customers and stakeholders and then selecting interventions that allow the service to meet those needs in the fastest, most cost-effective manner* (Dudden, 2007).

The emphasis is on the development and provision of resources and services to meet library customers' identified needs based on data rather than library staff's assumptions. In the past, library needs assessments generally were conducted with long-term comprehensive collection development in mind, yet with the rapid pace at which medical research is now being transformed into current practice, it's essential that consumer health collections and services are equally up to date in order to serve patrons' immediate information needs. Correspondingly, delivery mechanisms are continually evolving requiring assessment and benchmarking to ensure information delivery remains relevant. The benefits of needs assessment for collection development and services include:

- Increased likelihood for collections and services to meet customers' needs.
- Providing data for the allocation of existing or requested new resources.
- Providing data supporting existing or potential new services.
- Confirming that resources are serving the customers' needs.
- Providing service strategies for the customers' needs.
- Identifying and eliminating unneeded services and/or collections (Biblarz, Bosch, and Sugnet, 2001).

Conducting a Needs Assessment

Getting Started: Assessing Existing Resources and Defining Purpose

First, consider what capacity is available in terms of staff time, expertise, and resources. Does current staff have sufficient time to conduct the needs assessment? Can work duties be adjusted? Can other departments provide staff to assist? Does staff have experience with survey or questionnaire development, administration, and analysis, or is additional training required? Are circulation and website statistics of existing consumer health information collections available to consult for baseline data? Are staff familiar with the areas being assessed? Are existing resources (computers, phones, meeting rooms for focus groups, budget for print survey materials and postage) adequate or is additional funding needed (Biblarz, Bosch, and Sugnet, 2001)?

Next, review the organization's mission and vision statements; these can serve as a framework for identifying library user populations and the consumer health information resources and services needed to serve them. Ask other department administrators if recent environmental scans, SWOT analysis (internal Strengths and Weaknesses of the organization, external Opportunities and Threats of the environment), or related strategic planning has been done recently. This helps to better identify internal and external factors affecting the organization and associated consumer health information needs, such as increased awareness of health literacy and reading levels of patient education materials for a hospital. Further information about strategic planning for consumer health libraries is provided in Chapter 3 of this book.

It is helpful to focus on the broader community's health in addition to the internal and external factors affecting the organization in order to better understand the past, present, and potential future health status for the area. This includes identifying factors such as:

- Transportation infrastructure that does or doesn't support active communities (public transit, sidewalks, bicycling paths, grocery and other stores within walkable distance).
- Living environments that can affect health (low income and subpar housing developments with little access to community services, the presence of major industrial companies within residential neighborhoods).
- Insight from community culture (city mottos and slogans, behaviors that are encouraged or ignored such as domestic violence and drug abuse).
- Networking with existing organizations aware of community health needs such as service and advocacy groups, and community health clinics and hospitals (Work Group for Community Health and Development, 2012).

Bright Idea: For consumer health librarians in nonprofit hospitals, the organization's formal Community Health Needs Assessment (CHNA), required by the Affordable Care Act in concert with the Internal Revenue Service, provides invaluable information on the most pressing health needs of the community as well as a blueprint for addressing them. To the extent possible, consumer health librarians are encouraged to position their library resources to respond to the local CHNA's identified priorities as part of the larger strategic organizational response. Helpful resources to support CHNA work are available from the Centers for Disease Control and Prevention (Centers for Disease Prevention and Control, 2013).

Regardless of which approach is used, this in-depth information is then developed into a community health overview, which can be a brief summary of bullet points or a detailed report depending on your available resources. Such an overview provides important context and takes stock of the current health environment against which to measure progress made as a result of responding to identified needs with consumer health resources and services.

With the needs assessment team established and the organization and community's environment in mind, the project scope can then be defined. Will the needs assessment establish, update, reduce, and/or expand the library's consumer health information resources and services in general? Or will it target specific subject areas or user populations, such as patients with diabetes or seniors? By being as specific as possible in terms of the needs assessment's purposes and goals, the team will be able to identify relevant data to be collected. At this point in the planning process, the team leader will want to establish preliminary timelines: a due date for the project, and alignment with other projects, such as library strategic planning. These timelines will be further refined as the types of data for the needs assessment are identified.

What to Ask: Quantitative and Qualitative Data

Needs assessment does not necessarily mean creating a quick survey and expecting results to identify every possible consumer health information need. The first step is deciding whether the needs assessment will gather quantitative (primarily numeric) data, qualitative (primarily non-numeric) data, or possibly a combination of both.

The following figure from the Outreach Evaluation Resource Center of the National Network of Libraries of Medicine is one way to determine appropriate methodology.

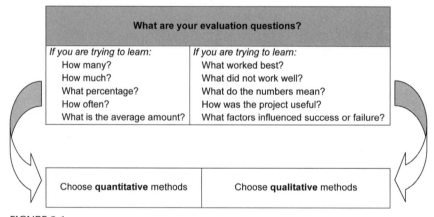

FIGURE 2.1
Choosing Type of Method (Olney and Barnes, 2013)

To describe in comprehensive detail all the processes involved for every type of quantitative and qualitative data collection method and data analysis is beyond the scope of this chapter. However, a general overview is given here to be instructive. The chapter bibliography provides resources for additional reference should more in-depth information be desired. In particular, the second edition of *Planning and Evaluating Health Information Outreach Projects* from the Outreach Evaluation Resource Center's website is a freely available and detailed resource that provides instruction for designing community consumer health information outreach programs, including assessment measures. The third booklet of the series, "Collecting and Analyzing Evaluation Data" (Olney and Barnes, 2013), is the source of the three figures included within this chapter. Additionally, this booklet includes helpful appendixes covering further quantitative and qualitative methods, along with toolkits containing worksheets for planning surveys and interviews.

Quantitative Data: Surveys

Needs assessment information obtained via user surveys is often more relevant for collection development and library service decisions than a review of circulation statistics, website hits, and other data sources. Depending upon the survey's scope, data obtained directly from patrons can assess their patterns of information usage, their knowledge of the available consumer health information resources at the library, and their understanding of consumer health information within the context of the library's broader organizational structure and community.

The benefits of surveys as needs assessment tools include the fact that survey results often precisely define individual information needs, and there is generally a high rate of statistical correlation of the data obtained, meaning that if users report they are satisfied with particular consumer health information resources or services provided by the library, they actually are happy with those services. Surveys also are opportunities to increase awareness of consumer health information resources and promote the library's services. Data gathered directly from users resonate strongly with administrators, who are more likely to allocate resources towards services that are clearly valued and desired by the community.

Nevertheless, be aware that survey development, administration, and assessment take a considerable amount of staff resources and expertise. This process takes time, and if other surveys have recently been administered by the library or organization, users may perceive they are being asked too frequently, leading to reduced participation and results of lesser quality (Biblarz, Bosch, and Sugnet, 2001).

The following figure provides a guide for designing surveys; collecting, summarizing and analyzing data; and assessing the validity of survey findings.

| Step 1 | **Design Your Data Collection Methods - Surveys** |

- Write your evaluation questions
- Develop the data collection tool (i.e., questionnaire)
- Pilot test the questionnaire

| Step 2 | **Collect Your Data - Surveys** |

- Decide who will receive the questionnaire
- Maximize response rate
- Check for nonresponse bias
- Provide motivation and information about risks and participants' rights

| Step 3 | **Summarize and Analyze Your Data** |

- Compile descriptive data
- Calculate measures of central tendency and dispersion
- Simplify data to explore trends
- Provide comparisons

| Step 4 | **Assess the Validity of Your Findings** |

- Calculate response rate
- Look for low completion rate of specific sections of surveys
- Investigate socially desirable responding

FIGURE 2.2
Steps to Develop and Assess Quantitative Data (Olney and Barnes, 2013)

When designing a needs assessment survey, good standards for high-quality questions will increase the likelihood of accurate, helpful responses. Some quality check areas include:

- Are the survey's instructions clear and easy to follow?
- Is the survey too brief or too long for the information being sought?

- Are the questions clear, using plain language and avoiding ambiguity?
- Do the questions rely heavily on the users' memory of seeking consumer health information?
- Are the questions too sensitive, asking users to reveal information that could be perceived as being of a highly personal nature?
- Is the survey designed so that the results can be coded or downloaded to data analysis programs easily and accurately? (Dudden, 2007)

Qualitative Data: Interviews

While qualitative data can also be obtained via surveys through the use of open-ended questions and text boxes, personal interviews and focus groups have proven to be reliable sources for identifying users' consumer health information needs and informing library services. When guided by qualitative methods, these tools can obtain valuable insights, opinions, and perspectives that would not be possible to collect solely through statistical data methods.

Focus groups are helpful when it's important to determine users' opinions about a planned service or collection development area. Focus groups usually consist of a small number (between seven to ten) of representative user subgroups, for example, parents of children with diabetes, who are assembled to discuss questions that have been provided to them well in advance, giving them time to consider their responses. The discussion is recorded with the participants' permission and guided by an experienced facilitator. It is important to keep in mind there is a high potential for bias because the focus group may not statistically represent a larger user population, yet the process can help clarify or correct assumptions library staff have regarding individuals and their consumer health information needs (Biblarz, Bosch, and Sugnet, 2001).

Another way to obtain qualitative opinion data from users is through the use of interviews, which are less formal than surveys and more conducive to individual responses than focus groups. Interviews follow a set of predetermined questions yet allow for personal interaction and additional clarifying questions. This process can provide richer results, leading to better understanding of consumer behaviors, needs, and interests in seeking library services.

The following figure provides a guide for designing questions, conducting interviews, summarizing and analyzing data, and assessing the validity of interview data.

| **Step 1** | **Design Your Data Collection Methods - Interviews** |

- Write your evaluation questions
- Develop the data collection tool (i.e. interview guide)
- Pilot test the interview guide

⇓

| **Step 2** | **Collect Your Data - Interviews** |

- Decide who will be interviewed
- Provide informed consent information
- Record the interviews
- Build trust and rapport through conversation
- Start the analysis during data collection

⇓

| **Step 3** | **Summarize and Analyze Your Data** |

- Prepare the text
- Note themes (or categories)
- Code the text
- Interpret results

⇓

| **Step 4** | **Assess the Trustworthiness of Your Findings** |

- Use procedures that check the fairness of your interpretations
- Present findings to reflect multiple points of view

FIGURE 2.3
Steps to Develop and Assess Qualitative Data (Olney and Barnes, 2013)

Participants are chosen for interviews through random sampling of users or through "key informant" interviews. Key informants are people "selected on the basis of criteria such as knowledge, compatibility, age, experience, or reputation who provide information about their culture. They can contribute a knowledgeable perspective on the nature and scope of a social problem or a target population. They know the community as a whole, or the particular portion the library is interested in learning more about. They can be professional persons, young or old, or from a variety of socioeconomic levels or ethnic groups" (Dudden, 2007, p. 312).

Interview questions are designed using the same methods as survey questions, each with a specific purpose in mind. As with pilot testing of surveys, having several test interviews with people who can offer feedback about the clarity of the questions is important before expanding to more individuals. Types of interview settings include in-person, telephone, and online methods using webcasting or video-casting.

Another important consideration is selecting the right interviewer. Interviewers must be highly skilled listeners and observers who do not interrupt conversations or talk too frequently. They should know how to guide conversations without dominating the discussion. Ideally, they would be members of the same user group from a demographic or other perspective to elicit candid responses, but if this isn't possible, the interviewer needs to be highly sensitive to the participants to avoid any potential for cultural misunderstandings or other misinterpretations. Plans should be made to obtain participants' permission to record the interviews, and for subsequent transcription.

Three types of needs assessment interviews are:

1. A standardized, open-ended interview where the same questions are asked in the same sequence among members of a sample population by different interviewers
2. Guided, structured interviews where the same questions are asked but opportunities for personal expression are allowed within a limited amount of time
3. The informal conversational interview where the interviewer can ask set questions yet is allowed the freedom to rapidly respond to users' replies

Each of these types of interviews can be helpful to obtain specific, focused answers that are easily comparable to broad insights, requiring more time for systematic analysis (Dudden, 2007).

Case Studies

The following case studies exemplify various approaches to needs assessments in consumer health libraries.

Case Study: Consumer Health Library Needs Assessment Work for a New Location

Mount Carmel Health Sciences Library in Columbus, Ohio, originally opened a three-hundred-square-foot consumer health library in March 2011 to serve patients on the second floor of a local nursing health center. In October 2013, the consumer health library reopened in a new location eight times larger (2,400 square feet) than the original location on the first floor next to a parking lot for patients. As part of both the establishment of the original consumer health library and again in preparation for moving into a greatly expanded space, needs assessment work was done in order to focus on what collection and services would be of optimal use for their patrons.

The collection in the original consumer health library location included between 100 and 130 monographs, which were mostly encyclopedias and other books containing anatomy images; anatomical models to explain conditions to patients and visitors including a complete torso, all organs, heart, knee, and hip; thirty DVDs of health conditions; and nineteen consumer health journal subscriptions. Library staff also worked with the patient education department, which provided the library with statistics about the diagnostic frequency of chronic diseases, and graduate students of Kent State University School of Library and Information Science on practicum assignments, to develop a large number of health pamphlets in order to meet the information needs of the nursing health center.

The library staff noticed that patrons were not often interested in using the books as resources, even with the availability of free library accounts and the ability to check out materials from the library. Instead, patrons expressed their appreciation for library staff assisting them at computers and teaching them how to search for and navigate online health information resources. MedlinePlus was the library's core online health information resource, with others including EBSCO's Consumer Health Complete, Healthy People 2020, Healthfinder.gov, and links to patient education material created internally for the nursing health center.

Before the consumer health library first opened in 2011, the library director conducted a study of Columbus area public libraries to assess the librarians' comfort level in providing health information and also to identify frequently asked health information questions and continuing health education needs. The results of this work provided the first foundational stone of the consumer health library by proving the need for professional staff librarians to manage consumer health information. The director then performed a community assessment, obtaining statistics that represented the socioeconomic status, education levels, common health issues, literacy, and related demographics of the area. The director worked very closely with local organizations to gain their user census data and obtain copies of their local survey results thereby avoiding duplication. He then based the consumer health library's resources and services on the information learned from these existing data resources.

The director next explored the consumer health needs for resident physicians in the hospital's clinics—specifically their time dedicated to patient education and what information resources the library could offer to help these efforts. As a result of this process, collaborative relationships were developed between clinicians and the consumer health library so patients didn't have to make return appointments with physicians to understand their diagnoses but were referred to the library for information services. Clear disclaimers indicated that library staff were not consulting with patients but providing information for them and their caregivers. Library staff took the time to sit and work with the many referred patients and caregivers who came to the consumer health library, often in emotional distress.

To help meet the needs of public librarians, Mount Carmel librarians encouraged them to refer patrons when more comprehensive information was needed, such as recovery information after a shoulder replacement surgery, and emphasized the need for patrons to talk with their physicians about the particulars of their surgical case, like details regarding their mobility and personal care plans.

As part of the needs assessment work for their new consumer health library, Mount Carmel staff visited other local consumer health libraries to conduct interviews and hold focus groups. Their goal was to learn more about what services these libraries provide for their patrons, what baseline information is used to establish their services and collection, and how they organize their workloads. Mount Carmel staff did not conduct or review existing surveys during this process as they wanted to spend the most time in the physical library environment, meeting face-to-face with people to help build networking relationships. To help staff determine what library services would best benefit the community, additional population analysis was done using locally available information, such as socioeconomic data from the United Way and health information literacy study results from the Ohio Department of Health.

The Mount Carmel director also met with the state librarian to determine what education programs the state library was planning for public and other librarians on providing consumer health information, and learned the state library couldn't organize these types of classes due to funding. The director then asked if the state library would be comfortable with Mount Carmel taking the initiative to offer this training as a nonprofit medical library in conjunction with funding and resources from the Medical Library Association and the National Network of Libraries of Medicine. They agreed upon this training initiative.

The director also established a partnership with a local assisted living community, where the facility provided space and allowed the Mount Carmel consumer health library staff to promote their services there.

With the reopening of the Mount Carmel consumer health library in 2013, staff continue to collaborate with local organizations and public libraries, offering their collective resources to serve the people in the community. Library staff practice within the community, such as having displays at health fairs and at an international festival where free flu vaccinations are offered, providing information about vaccines in seven to ten different languages. The library now offers more interactive activities, including space to promote healthy eating by organizing cooking classes for health conditions such as diabetes. These classes help people increase awareness of their health conditions and change their eating habits. In addition to continuing to use the same online health information resources, the library continues seeking new resources that are provided by government, nonprofit organizations, and others in support of open access. They are grouped together by themes on their website for easier access and navigation.

In planning the new consumer health library, the director didn't feel pressure to meet established library standards and wanted to make the new consumer health library comfortable, open, and homelike, so patrons would feel a sense of belonging. The facility is compliant with the American Disabilities Act (ADA), with a large display housing their five hundred health information pamphlets as an integral part of a wall design. The new library does not have large bookshelves due to their minimal use of monographs. They designed a lively children's area with coloring activities, a television playing cartoon shows, and computers with children's Internet filters to occupy them while their parents and caregivers use the rest of the library's resources. There is a privacy room for library staff consultations with emotionally distressed patrons or for discussing patrons' sensitive health information. This room is secluded with dimmed glass so that passersby can't see in. The library is currently advocating for a larger television screen for a marketing display as its current monitor is too small for seniors to easily read the display information. It seeks to be seen as a place that accommodates all community needs and welcomes everyone, from those patrons seeking health information to those just checking their email or simply in need of a comfortable place to sit and relax (Roksandic, 2013).

Case Study: Library Website Needs Assessment Work with Consumer Health Information

During the 2013 Washington Medical Librarians Association (http://www.wmla.org) meeting, Christa Werle presented the process followed by the Sno-Isle Libraries' System to redesign its website to make their resources, including consumer health information, easier for users to find. Some of the factors driving their needs assessment were:

- The changing scope of reference questions (including consumer health topics) to more in-depth inquiries
- To provide both the justification and relevance for continued library funding
- A desire to build relationships with other library departments, such as Information Technology and Administration
- To work with third-party vendors to better locate their content on the library's website

Initially, in 2010, the Sno-Isle Libraries' website contained thirty subject categories with more than one thousand recommended links. This was reduced to 150 recommended websites in 2012, and when web metrics were checked, the library learned the recommended websites had no usage at all. Studying a combination of the libraries' data points such as QuestionPoint online chat service, website comments and questions, staff input, technical reports, and related feedback channels, fourteen recurring user themes were identified. Themes included the need for adding video tutorials and vendor user guides to resources, highlighting the libraries' top ten databases by usage, using more images and graphics to list subject categories and resources, and simplifying any text on the website to fifteen words or fewer. Results of a usability study showed customers didn't have a clear sense of direction on the website: users needed information immediately but couldn't find it.

Sno-Isle Libraries established a staff team including "big picture thinkers" and "doers," and developed a clear sense of purpose: their goal was to redesign the website to meet their audiences' online information needs. The next step was identifying the website's audiences, which were not the one hundred Sno-Isle librarians and all 672,000 members of the public living in the surrounding counties, but more focused subgroups of who the libraries were trying to reach with their information resources. To survey their target audiences, they publicized frequently using a variety of communication channels (website ads, emails, social media mentions). The team also reviewed what information was being accessed on the website along with information they knew was missing or misplaced, such as high-interest, existing content areas that patrons nevertheless couldn't locate.

Next, the team considered and discussed areas of emphasis such as:

- What information had to be maintained?
- Which pages generated the most website traffic?
- Were there any new content themes to address?
- How would they prioritize information?
- Was there anything to discard?

The team then worked with their website designers to clarify what parts of the webpage *couldn't* be changed, such as headers and footers. One way the team brainstormed how to arrange its website content was to use big sheets of paper as a blank slate to explore ways to fill in the detail. There might not have been total consensus, but a majority decision sufficed.

In order to generate concrete and specific ideas for website topic development, staff printed blue cards of existing topic areas to identify their priorities. The next step was sorting website categories into themes, and in this process the staff was able to narrow thirty-four subject categories to twelve. With the twelve subject categories defined, the staff then limited themselves to three to five recommended websites per content section.

The team then sent their work to the designers and received website prototypes. During their subsequent review, preferences quickly became apparent, but these may reflect past habits and tendencies; so, it was essential to crosscheck these preferences with what the users said they really wanted.

Next, everyone gathered for a final review team meeting, including the content creators and designer. They considered how often the team would want to revisit the website design with more usability studies or another outreach campaign, keeping in mind that future efforts are often limited by staff time and budget.

Effectiveness of website revisions and redesign in meeting users' consumer health information needs is best determined through actual usage: if baseline data were collected, the needs assessment team would be able to compare whether their intended goals are being achieved and whether "funnels" for user behavior (such as the process to request an interlibrary loan of a consumer health monograph) are being used. If there are no baseline data, it would be difficult for the team to accurately assess improvement. Note: there are free programs such as Google Analytics, and many content management systems that have built-in analytics, but it's not enough just to keep up the account without investing time to understand the functionality of the program, what types of data it can generate, and how to download data for analysis.

The Sno-Isle Libraries Research page, where consumer health information resources are now consolidated under the Healthy Living subject area, had an increase in usage of 62.8 percent after the needs assessment and website redesign. Future challenges for the website include justifying its relevancy for continued funding, the library's role in increasing awareness of digital literacy, and continuing to build relationships with the Information Technology department for support. Opportunities for Sno-Isle Libraries include ways to increase accessibility of its information for users with mobile devices, including responsive design that is scalable to different screen sizes by chunking the website content information into accessible pieces (Werle, 2013).

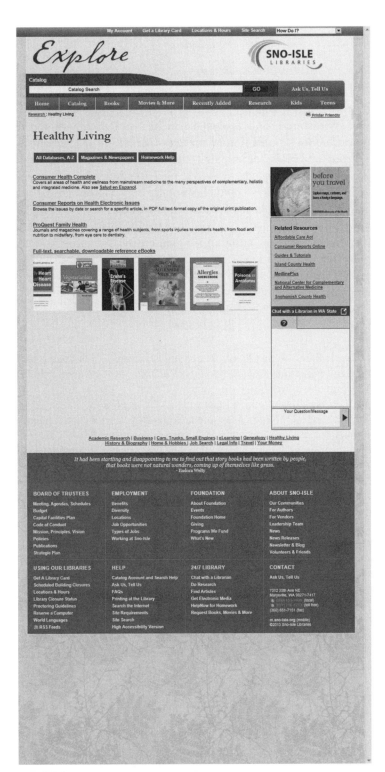

FIGURE 2.4
Sno-Isle Libraries Consumer Health Information Website

Conclusion

In addition to strategic planning, a needs assessment that is well planned, designed, administered, and analyzed can be the benchmark for future collection development and library services. An additional benefit is that library patrons and stakeholders are given an opportunity to directly express their information needs, which is vital to library budget planning. Tangible data gained in a systematic fashion through surveys, focus groups, interviews, and other tools are critical for budgeting (Silver, 2004). At a broader level, they offer persuasive evidence to administrators and the general public that the library is not an isolated entity, but rather a vital part of the collective organization, with its own unique role in advancing the organization's mission.

References

Biblarz, D, Bosch, S, and Sugnet, C, eds. 2001. *Guide to Library User Needs Assessment for Integrated Information Resource Management and Collection Development*. Lanham, MD: Scarecrow Press.

Centers for Disease Prevention and Control. 2013. "Resources for Implementing the Community Health Needs Assessment Process." Last modified September 13, 2013. http://www.cdc.gov/policy/chna/. Accessed November 1, 2013.

Dey, A. 2004. "Consumer Health Informatics: An Overview of Patient Perspectives on Health Information Needs." *The HIM Journal*, 33(4):121–26.

Dudden, RF. 2007. *Using Benchmarking, Needs Assessment, Quality Improvement, Outcome Measurement, and Library Standards*. How-To-Do-It Manuals for Librarians Number 159.

Olney, CA, and Barnes, SJ. 2013. "Collecting and Analyzing Evaluation Data, 2nd Edition." National Network of Libraries of Medicine. http://guides.nnlm.gov/oerc_tools. Accessed May 13, 2013.

Roksandic, S (Mount Carmel Library Director), in discussion with the author, August 2013.

Werle, C. 2013. "Streamline Content for Your Users & You: Content Strategy for Sustainable Site Maintenance." WMLA Annual Meeting 2013 Conference Presentation, July 12, 2013, Bastyr University, Seattle, Washington.

Work Group for Community Health and Development. 2012. "Chapter 3: Assessing Community Needs and Resources." *Community Toolbox*. Lawrence: University of Kansas. http://ctb.ku.edu/en/tablecontents/chapter_1003.aspx. Accessed October 28, 2013.

3

Strategic Planning for Success

Mary Grace Flaherty

Introduction

CAREFUL PLANNING IS OFTEN AN essential element to maximize the potential success of any new project, product, or service. There are numerous approaches and extensive literature devoted to strategic planning, mostly borne out of corporate and business models and experiences (see, for instance, Barnes, 2011; Calonius, 2011; Fry, Stoner, and Weinzimmer, 2005; Govindarajan and Trimble, 2012; Kates, 2012; Lafley and Martin, 2013). A common theme in many of these approaches is responsiveness to the user (insert the term applied to your audience here, for example, customer, patient, or patron, etc.) of the product or service while keeping a clear vision of and commitment to the organization's overall mission.

Consumer health information provision can take place and is taking place in a wide variety of library or information service settings, including but not limited to hospitals or clinics, academic settings, statewide or regional library systems or consortia, as well as special, public, and school libraries. Of course, each setting will be unique with regard to organizational structure and function, but for planning purposes, there are commonalities across all of these settings.

The Parent Organization

The institutional or organizational setting of the consumer health library is an important consideration and will play a major role in how services are delivered. Whether the consumer health library or resource is located in a multi-tiered national healthcare system or a standalone public library will have a profound effect on how strategic planning is carried out, though some elements are likely to be similar, if not the same. In the multi-tiered setting, there will presumably be a longer timeline with more players to involve and bring on board while in settings such as the small hospital or special library, the director and/or staff may have greater autonomy with regard to formulating and adopting new service provision. In settings such as public libraries, an appointed or elected library board of trustees may exert a great deal of influence on service and policy changes. Sometimes strategic planning is geared towards a specific issue or goal, such as increasing funding or external resources (Gall, Lilly, and Miller, 1997). In any setting, an important first step is to ensure the service or goal fits in with the overall mission of the parent organization.

The Mission Statement

Mission statements are characterized as official statements of organizations or businesses that describe their basic purpose or overall aim. An effective mission statement should:

- Define what the library does.
- Specify who uses the resource.
- Identify benefits of using the library.
- Focus on the present.
- Be brief, and clearly written without acronyms or buzzwords (Matthews, 2005).

Additionally, the library's mission statement should be in keeping with and reflect the goals and expectations of the parent organization or institution. As part of the strategic planning process, the mission statement should be reviewed to be certain it accurately reflects the overarching organizational purpose and goals. Once the planning process is complete, the mission statement should be revisited periodically and revised as needed.

Planning: Where to Start?

The planning process is likely to differ somewhat depending upon whether the organization is focused on creating a new consumer health information service or revising or adapting an already established service. Perhaps a renovation to the physical facility or increased funding through grants or a bequest allows for new dedicated space and/or funds for the service, or a change in administration has opened up opportunities for new priorities. Most organizations engage in long-range and strategic planning that envelop much more than just one service, but for the sake of illustration, this discussion will focus on the service of providing consumer health information in the context of the larger organizational setting.

Establishing Services: Starting from Scratch

Imagine a senior leader walks into the office of the library director and asks for a presentation of a preliminary strategic plan for providing consumer health information at the next general organizational meeting. Where should the library director start? Who should be involved in the process? What are some of the elements to consider? How is a strategic plan different from other types of planning documents?

A strategic plan is one type of tool that organizations utilize to achieve their mission. An effective strategic plan should specify goals, action steps, and the resources needed to achieve the goals. It should be reviewed at least every three to five years. An organization's operating plan is usually a one-year plan and will be more detailed than a strategic plan. It more thoroughly spells out the steps or tasks needed to achieve the goals in the strategic plan, with a delineation of staff duties and specific timelines (Mittenthal, 2002). To begin the process of creating a strategic plan, some initial considerations and elements are included in the following.

Aspects of the Strategic Plan

- Does the new service fit within the organization's mission?
  - Review mission statements for the library and its parent organization.
  - Define the service's audience (public, hospital patients, etc.).
- Determine where the library is presently, and where the library would like to be with regard to provision of services.
  - Set preliminary goals (broad goals at first, for example, creating consumer health information resource center or outreach to a new community of users).
- Identify key players and stakeholders.
  - Be strategic—include advocates as well as individuals who may not be keen supporters.
  - Look beyond the immediate department or organization for input.
  - Include staff from different organizational levels.

- ○ Assure that individuals can make the necessary effort and time commitment.
- Establish what resources are available (not only for the planning process, but for providing and promoting the service or resource).
  - ○ Physical facility.
  - ○ Funding.
  - ○ Staffing.
  - ○ Materials and other resources in a variety of formats (e.g., electronic resources, print, programming, etc.).
  - ○ Identify other possible funding sources (e.g., small grants, foundations, local businesses, etc.).
- Fine-tune goals.
  - ○ Refine and create specific goals.
  - ○ Ensure they are realistic.
  - ○ Get buy-in from stakeholders.
  - ○ Identify measurable objectives for each goal (e.g., if providing programs is one of the agreed-upon specific goals: *By this date, the library will host x amount of programs related to health issues.*).
- Identify strategies and action plans for completing goals and objectives.
- Determine timeline.
  - ○ Ensure it is realistic.
  - ○ Build in a cushion for unforeseen circumstances (e.g., construction or hiring/staffing delays).
- Provide process for review, assessment, evaluation, and follow-up.
  - ○ Regularly review the goals and objectives.
  - ○ Revisit strategic plan and revise as needed.
- Plan for sustainability.
  - ○ Establish where and how the service fits into the larger organizational structure and function.
  - ○ Determine how the service will continue (e.g., staff, funding, resource provision, etc.).

Bright Lights: During the planning process, sound approaches to help maximize the likelihood of success include the following:

Keep the lines of communication open.
Keep stakeholders apprised of your progress with regular updates.
Make regular assessments and reports of progress towards goals.
Don't be afraid to make changes and adapt as needed.
Celebrate accomplishments along the way.

Strategic planning is a process rather than an endpoint. By incorporating an assessment component, through elements such as measurable objectives and specified timelines, the organization can track progress towards the goals that were determined at the start of the process. Of course, it is likely there will be unforeseen circumstances and changes, so adaptability and flexibility are necessary during this and all other phases of the planning process, as well as a good dose of common sense. Keep track of what is working, and adapt services as necessary. For example, if users aren't turning to print materials, consider downsizing the print collection and offering a greater variety of alternative formats. If one of the goals is to increase patronage, then reach out to the community of nonusers to determine how the library can serve their needs; consider expanding into programs on health promotion and other activities. For instance, if there's a daycare center for staff at the facility, deliver and provide materials there on parenting or child care that staff can use. Perhaps the library can propose hosting a weekly storytime hour to promote library services as well.

Strategic planning doesn't happen in a vacuum. Consumer health information settings are not unique in a common and primary requirement for survival—no matter if the entity is an organization, service, or product— that is, remaining relevant to communities of users, whoever and wherever they may be. Thus, library staff should get out into the organizational, institutional, and greater communities to find out how they can serve their users, and identify those groups of users that they may not be reaching. Formal data gathering mechanisms, such as surveys and focus groups or interviews, can help to supply this information. Less formal mechanisms and anecdotal data can also be meaningful for collecting information about user communities. Library staff can take advantage of informal opportunities, such as waiting in the lunch line or riding on the elevator to engage users, simply by asking them if they know about the library or service. If they don't, this is an opportunity to educate them, and ask how they can be motivated to use the library (or to attend programs, etc.). In planning and building the library of the future, there are two critical components to consider: a focus on users' changing needs and the role of the library as a service rather than a collection (Stoffle and Cuillier, 2011).

Of course, it would be great to have a magic crystal ball at one's disposal when it comes to future projections and how the library should be positioned to meet changing needs and demands for service. As this resource is not likely to be available, other tools for prognostication, such as census predictions, county data, and demographic assessments can be used. For example, is the community attracting retirees or new immigrants? If so, this will have an impact on the strategic planning process and library services. In healthcare settings, data on diagnosis-related groups can also impart information on health status and prevalent conditions of resource users. Using this type of data can help to inform the planning process and subsequent service provision.

The following examples are composites of consumer health information services taking place in a variety of library settings, in order to illustrate the role of planning in "real world" settings.

Example: Consumer Health Services in an Urban Hospital Setting

Just One Piece of the Pie

In this large urban hospital facility, a major renovation and construction of a new children's center allowed for the creation of a patient/consumer health information center geared primarily towards pediatric patients and their families/caregivers. Because the facility is part of a state-supported academic research facility, it is required to be open to the public. At the time of the renovation, the hospital had a well-established health sciences library, used mostly by clinical staff and medical students. The director of the health sciences library was included in the long-range and strategic planning of a patient information center in the new children's center. His input was geared towards issues such as how to arrange the facility, what resources to provide, and the hiring of new staff. As part of a much larger organization, his input was very targeted, though vital to the day-to-day function and operation of the information center.

One of his main concerns, which he voiced at meetings throughout the planning phase, was admittance for visitors, especially because of state re- quirements for public access to resources. The patient information center is located on the fifteenth floor, and in order to gain entry one must register with a guard before getting on an elevator, creating a barrier and thus hindering, maybe even discouraging, access. There wasn't much room for negotiation on this point, as the location of the patient information center was predetermined at a much earlier stage in the planning process. In order to compensate, the library director ensured visible signage with clear instructions on how to get into the center were posted in the lobby entrances throughout the new chil- dren's center and hospital. This example demonstrates the importance of the library director having a seat at the table early on in the larger organization's strategic planning process. If he had been included in the preliminary phases of planning, he could have voiced his concerns as space allocations were being determined and made the pitch to locate the patient information center in a more accessible setting, such as on the first floor.

Example: Consumer Health Information Services
in a Suburban Public Library

Sometimes Opportunity Knocks without a Plan

In this case, little actual strategic or organizational planning took place; provision of consumer health information was encompassed in the library's services through motivated staff and a supportive organizational and institutional structure and atmosphere. In this suburban public library, an innovative staff member completed the Consumer Health Information Specialization (CHIS) credential through the Medical Library Association, largely due to her personal interest in the area. A few years later, her supervisor asked her to be interviewed by the local newspaper to publicize consumer health information as a library service. At that time, a reporter interviewed her, asked for specific examples, and published a piece in the front section of the local newspaper that received considerable attention in the community.

The staff member then took the opportunity to create a more visible consumer health resource for patrons in her community. She took a corner of unused space in the library and transferred the health reference collection there. Now the area includes three full bookshelves and a table for newsletters and brochures—some are free, some are subscriptions (e.g., *Harvard Women's Health, Berkeley Wellness, MedlinePlus* magazine, etc.). Many of the items in the health reference collection have been transferred to standing orders. The library gives periodic reminders to the public about the service, and two dedicated, CHIS-trained staff members compile, on average, between three to five very detailed consumer health information packets for individual patrons every month. The consumer health services effort has won recognition from the state and regional library system. According to annual report data, the library answers approximately sixty thousand reference questions annually (New York State Division of Library Development, 2012), and library staff estimate that 15 to 20 percent of those reference questions are health related. Notebooks with a record of each consumer health reference encounter are kept, and this information helps to guide collection development in the area of health.

As the service has evolved, the library now hosts many health-related programs and engages in collaborative relationships within the larger community (including local healthcare providers, hospitals, nonprofits, etc.). Programs are usually very well attended, including a Lyme disease support group that meets every month with about sixty to seventy attendees. Local partnerships include a local care center's mobile mammography van set up in the library's parking lot, filling every appointment; a hospital that provides resources such as free screenings; a breast cancer education organization that provides information and programs; individual healthcare providers who give presentations on subjects such as autism, nutrition, etc.; and other non-profit organizations (e.g., Planned Parenthood) who also provide information and programs. These relationships in the community have evolved over time through the efforts of engaged staff members.

In this example, CHIS was initiated by one individual. While the staff member did receive organizational support to attend CHIS classes as well as positive feedback from the library director and board, the service and the center were established with little planning and with the resources that were readily on hand. These unfunded efforts with outreach to the healthcare community have served to create a resource that is well utilized and appreciated by local citizens. This example illustrates that sometimes successful initiatives occur without extensive planning, but through the efforts of dedicated, motivated staff members with ongoing institutional and organizational support.

Conclusion

The amount of influence and input an individual will have in the strategic planning process within an organization or larger institution will vary, depending upon the institutional structure, culture, and setting. In larger organizational settings where the library is one component, it is important to create, maintain, and sustain relationships within the organization and larger community in order to remain highly visible. Doing so increases the likelihood that the department will be invited to be involved in the strategic planning process from the start. Strong partnerships and affiliations both within the organization and the community-at-large are not only essential, but are central to the success of the strategic planning process as well as the welfare of the library or organization. Through building and maintaining relationships, the library will remain viable and responsive to its community of users while fulfilling the organization's mission.

TABLE 3.1
Selected Resources for Developing a Strategic Plan

California State University Sacramento, *IT Strategic Planning*: http://www.csus.edu/irt/ cio/strategicplanning/documents/ITSPStrategicPlanning.pdf

Managance Consulting, *Sample Strategic Plan: The ABC Service Agency*: http://www .ecdcus.org/What_We_Do/Sample_StrategicPlan-ServiceAgency.pdf

Planware Organization, *Strategic Plan for AnyBiz, Inc.*: http://www.planware.org/ strategicsample.htm

Southwestern Association of Episcopal Schools, *Sample Strategic Plan*: http://www .swaes.org/Documents/strategic_plan.pdf

University of California Berkeley, *Strategic Planning Tip Sheet*: http://socrates.berkeley .edu/~pbd/pdfs/Strategic_Planning.pdf

U.S. General Services Administration, *Sample Strategic Plan, Community Child Development Center*: http://www.gsa.gov/graphics/pbs/Sample_Board_of_Director_ Strategic_Plan.pdf

TABLE 3.2
Sample Strategic Library Plans

Boston University Libraries: http://www.bu.edu/library/about/strategic-plan/

California State Library: http://www.library.ca.gov/about/cslstatplan.html

Carnegie Library of Pittsburgh: http://www.carnegielibrary.org/about/strategicplan/

Cornell University Library: http://www.library.cornell.edu/aboutus/inside/ strategicplanning

DeKalb County (Georgia) Public Library: http://www.dekalblibrary.org/newsflashes/ dekalb-county-public-library-s-strategic-plan.html

Duke University: http://library.duke.edu/about/planning/2010-2012/

Galter Health Sciences Library of Northwestern University: http://www.galter .northwestern.edu/images/cms/Libdocs/strategic_plan0812.pdf

Harvey Cushing/John Hay Whitney Medical Library of Yale University School of Medicine: http://doc.med.yale.edu/about/action2009.pdf

Seattle Public Library: http://www.spl.org/Documents/about/strategic_plan.pdf

University of North Carolina Health Sciences Library: http://hsl.lib.unc.edu/strategicplan

Vancouver Public Library: http://www.youtube.com/watch?v=Hi2cdSvgwPw

References

Barnes, B. 2011. *Everything I Know about Business I Learned from the Grateful Dead*. New York: Hachette Book Group.

Calonius, E. 2011. *Ten Steps Ahead*. New York: Penguin.

Fry, FL, Stoner, CR, and Weinzimmer, LG. 2005. *Strategic Planning for Small Business Made Easy*. Madison, WI: Entrepreneur Press.

Gall, CF, Lilly, R, and Miller, EG. 1997. "Strategic Planning with Multitype Libraries in the Community: A Model with Extra Funding as the Main Goal." *Bulletin of the Medical Library Association*, 85(3):252–59.

Govindarajan, V, and Trimble, C. 2012. *Reverse Innovation*. Boston, MA: Harvard Business Review Press.

Kates, A. 2012. *Find Your Next*. New York: McGraw-Hill.

Lafley, AG, and Martin, RL. 2013. *Playing to Win: How Strategy Really Works*. Boston, MA: Harvard Business Review Press.

Matthews, JR. 2005. *Strategic Planning and Management for Library Managers*. Westport, CT: Libraries Unlimited.

Mittenthal, RA. 2002. *Ten Keys to Successful Strategic Planning for Nonprofit and Foundation Leaders*. Briefing Paper. New York: TCC Group.

New York State Division of Library Development. 2012. *Bibliostat*. August 15, 2012. http://www.nysl.nysed.gov/libdev/libs/index.html. Accessed August 15, 2012.

Stoffle, CJ, and Cuillier, C. 2011. "From Surviving to Thriving." *Journal of Library Administration*, 51:130–55.

4

Bricks and Mortar:
Costs, Budgeting, and Funding

Cara Marcus

Introduction

EFFECTIVE BUDGETING IS A CRUCIAL, ongoing process for managers of consumer health information services. Sometimes a center will have its own budget or it may be part of a department or division within an organization. Patient education may be the responsibility of all providers, and components of the program may come from various budgets, such as the division of nursing and the community relations department (Rykwalder, 1987).

Creating a program budget is entirely different from balancing a personal checkbook. Library professionals new to the budget process should learn from their predecessors or managers how the budget is structured and prepared, and what existing software, training, and support are available.

Overview—Budgeting 101

Which type of budget should be used? Table 4.1 describes the most common budget models used in business settings.

Even if everyone else is using a line item budget, a patient education manager may use formula spreadsheets to track expenditures related to usage. Using multiple budget formats may be helpful and even necessary.

Budgets are generally divided into capital and operational components. Many organizations set thresholds for capital purchases, such as costs higher than five thousand dollars, which may require senior-level approval. Even

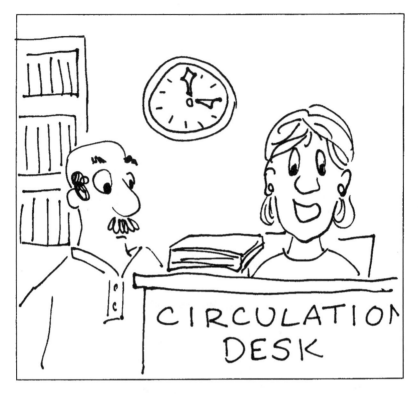

Your book is five years, two months and three days overdue. Let's see, that will be $1,281.55. But the good news is – now the library can buy a new computer.

FIGURE 4.1
Original Cartoon by Cara Marcus

TABLE 4.1
Budget Types

Name	Definition	Description	Issues and Challenges
Lump sum	A single amount of money is provided for the year to cover all the consumer health information service's financial needs. This is known as the "bottom line."	The manager is responsible for tracking and allocating funds. As long as the consumer health information service does not exceed the budget, the manager can spend where is most needed. When the allotted amount is reached, additional spending may need to wait until the next fiscal year.	This budget is often used if a consumer health library or patient education program is considered a line under another department's budget. Accurate record-keeping is very important to justify spending and requests for additional funding.
Formula	Costs are allocated to mathematical formulas related to numbers.	An example would be estimating the interlibrary loan (ILL) budget using the previous year's data of forty-two articles borrowed at an average cost of $11 each, for a total of $462, and setting an ILL budget line of $500 for the next year.	This type of budget does not account for unexpected expenses, such as book replacement after flooding, or new initiatives, such as starting an eBook collection.
Line item	Each line in the budget corresponds to an object code, usually set by the finance or accounting department of the parent organization.	There may be a line for subscriptions, supplies, computer hardware, computer software, etc.	Most accounting software systems are set up for line item budgets. The line item budget can use a formula that takes last year's costs and applies a 7 percent inflation increase to create line amounts for the next year's budget. New initiatives need to be requested and approved.

(continued)

TABLE 4.1
(continued)

Name	Definition	Description	Issues and Challenges
Program/performance/ function	Services associated with costs, such as document delivery, collection development, technical services, education, etc., are given lines rather than objects, such as books, brochures, magazines, etc.	Line item costs can be listed within each program/performance/function. Future cost estimates are based on historical data for costs in each area.	A program budget is more time consuming and challenging to develop than a simple line item budget. It's hard to accurately determine the percentage of supplies (staples, tape, etc.) that a library will use for classes as opposed to literature packets.
Zero-based	The budget is expected to remain at the same level of funding as the previous year or at a level determined by the organization.	The budget must be built from the same funding levels each year and every purchase needs to be justified.	This type of budget is one of the hardest to set up and manage, as resource costs usually increase each year, especially publications and subscriptions.
Capital	A capital budget is reserved for large physical purchases not in the regular budget, such as buildings, furniture, and computers.	This type of budget would be used to start a new consumer health information service or add new physical components. Capital requests usually have to be above a certain dollar amount and approved by senior management or the board.	As capital budgets are by nature much larger than annual operating budgets, and based on substantial one-time costs, they require coordination between many parties, such as planning committees, senior leadership, boards, development officers, architects, contractors, etc.

virtual consumer health services may require capital funding, as computers are often considered capital expenditures.

Operational budgets are used for day-to-day needs (resources, supplies, subscriptions, etc.). Personnel may be considered part of the operational budget. Large costs, such as databases, are often accrued over the year, so a twelve thousand dollar charge will not hit the budget in one month, but be spaced out in one thousand dollar monthly increments. Software can accomplish this "behind the scenes" and includes reports so managers can compare budgeted and actual spending (variances), monthly spending, year-to-date costs, line item costs, etc.

Managers use budget codes or cost centers to apply funds from their operational budget and may be able to pay by purchase order/requisition, check request, procurement/debit/credit card, electronic funds transfer, or a combination. Vendors send quotations for approval and invoices for payment. Accounts are set up for purchasing categories, including a miscellaneous account for items that do not fit into predefined categories.

Many libraries, hospitals, schools, etc., have nonprofit standing, which entitles them to tax-exempt status. Their consumer health information service is not required to pay sales tax on purchases, but needs to provide vendors official forms showing their tax exempt status and/or taxpayer identification number.

Budget Management Software and Tools

Budget tools range from simple ledger books and spreadsheets, such as Microsoft Excel, to software like Intuit Quicken, IBM Cognos, and numerous others. Excel can be used on most computers, including Macintosh and Hewlett Packard. Many integrated online library systems contain budgeting features that assist in tracking expenditures (Bandy and Dudden, 2011).

Desirable features in budget software are user friendliness, compatibility with other software, built-in budget assumption tools (such as inflation factors), and customizability. However, an organization may use a single tool and managers may not have a choice of software. If a manager can select budget software, he or she should contact other consumer health information specialists for recommendations, and contact vendors and request quotes, demonstrations, and trials.

Estimating Costs

New Consumer Health Information Centers and Initiatives

Consumer health information centers have different needs from public or even medical libraries. A budget for a new center includes all capital and

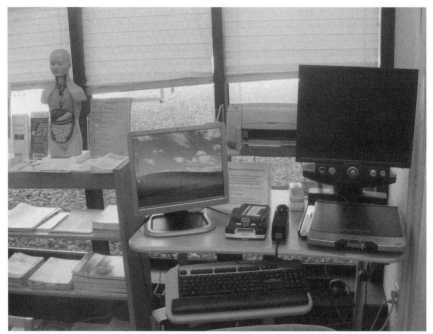

FIGURE 4.2
Photograph of Library Technology and Equipment

initial operational expenditures, including personnel, construction, equipment, and resource costs. Money often comes from a combination of sources including the parent organization and a fundraising campaign. When the Maxwell & Eleanor Blum Patient and Family Learning Center was established, both operational and capital funds were committed to build and staff it. Positions were approved for funding, and personnel were hired (Pittman, O'Connor, Millar, and Erickson, 2001).

Consumer health information centers are dynamic entities and must grow and embrace the new to provide the best services for patients and families. The manager should actively seek new technologies, services, and resources to enhance the program. New initiatives usually need to be justified in terms of cost-benefit to the parent organization.

Fiscal Years and Timelines

Fiscal years sometimes coincide with calendar years, but may run on a different cycle, like October through September. Budget deadlines are based on

TABLE 4.2
Timeline for an October to September Budget

January	Compile usage and cost data for previous year
February	Contact vendors for pricing
March	Draft budget
April	Submit final budget for manager approval
May	If budget is returned to you with any changes, adjust the final budget
June	Compile lists of resources (books, pamphlets, etc.) to purchase
July	Request renewal quotes from subscription vendors
August	Request quotes from book vendors
September	Order final materials from this year's budget—try to use entire amount
October	Begin the new budget—pay subscription vendors and begin to order other materials
November	Collection development—explore vendors and resource options
December	Schedule time for trainings, vendor demos, etc.

the fiscal year cycle. If the fiscal year begins in October, a manager may have to submit the budget for approval as early as April. A timeline is important for meeting deadlines, such as contacting vendors for fee estimates. Managers should allow at least one month for quotes.

Ongoing data collection is crucial for effective budgeting. To determine how many pamphlets a center needs each year, the staff should take an inventory of how many were used. Data collection can take place on a regular schedule (monthly, quarterly, or annually) or incrementally (adding costs of pamphlets purchased each day to a spreadsheet).

Table 4.2 shows a simple timeline that can be used to plan for budget deadlines.

Determining Consumer Health Information Center Needs

Determining which resources and programs will be provided guides the budget. Conducting a formal needs assessment; visiting or contacting other centers with questions; using professional organization lists, wikis, and blogs; and asking people within the organization what resources the consumer health information service should carry are recommended strategies. For hospital programs, service lines may guide decisions to order materials to support them. Resources and programs should be aligned with the consumer health information center's mission, vision, and goals. See Chapter 2 for an in-depth discussion of needs assessment.

There are no standards regarding types, formats, or number of resources a consumer health information service should provide. Budget constraints set a limit on what to buy initially. Available shelving and storage space also affect purchasing.

Types of Expenses

Books

Consumer health books cost less than medical textbooks, usually fifteen to fifty dollars (a few major textbooks are recommended, too, which can cost fifty to six hundred dollars). An average consumer health library carries between fifty and three hundred books. They don't all have to be purchased immediately! Managers need to budget for replacing lost or stolen books and purchasing new editions. Consumer health books usually get updated every three to five years. Vendors often offer approval plans which ship or notify managers about new editions.

Many consumer health books are now available in eBook format, for reading on computers and/or handheld devices, such as Kindle, Nook, iPad, and others. Libraries offering eBooks may need to purchase handheld readers, which are usually one to two hundred dollars each. There are free eBooks,

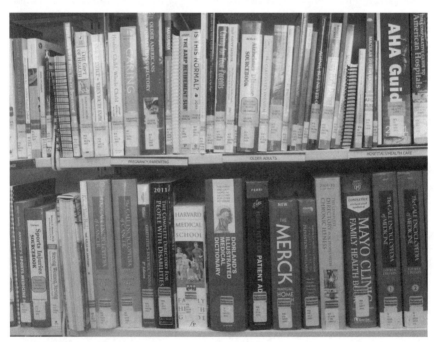

FIGURE 4.3
Photograph of Books on Library Shelf

> **Bright Idea:** Books can be purchased online from a book distribution company at a discounted rate, or a discount or used bookstore. Used books are available from large distributors, such as Amazon.com, and many other sellers. A "good as new" copy of a book is often available for as little as one dollar and is fine as long as it is the latest edition.

and some library systems offer free eBooks to their members, but generally eBooks cost the same or more than print books. Some vendors charge more for eBooks available to multiple readers. Large eBook collections are available through preselected vendor packages typically starting at one thousand dollars, with hundreds to thousands of titles. Once an eBook is purchased, similar to its print counterpart, the library owns it forever and is responsible for weeding it or purchasing the updated edition.

A patron-driven acquisition model is a new way to purchase eBooks, meaning the library purchases the books specifically requested by users, although research on this model has focused on large academic institutions and studies need to be done regarding its applicability to consumer health collections (Reiners, 2012).

Magazines and Newsletters

Some magazines and newsletters are free, but others usually cost about ten to one hundred dollars per year. Ten to forty subscriptions are about average. Using a subscription vendor may result in higher costs per title, plus service fees, but the benefits include simplified billing and the ability to claim issues not received. There are also many eMagazines and eNewsletters, which are often free.

It pays to shop around for a subscription vendor and request quotes, as costs vary. The center's budget cycle may not dovetail with publishers' cost increase cycle. Managers should expect and plan for potential cost increases of 5 to 10 percent per year, but may not know the final subscription costs until after the renewals have been approved.

Librarians may also want to budget for professional titles, including *Library Journal, Journal of Consumer Health on the Net, Searcher*, and others to assist with collection development, continuing education, and professional development.

Pamphlets and Brochures

Pamphlets are available from government agencies, vendors, and organizations. Many organizations now offer their free pamphlets online only, which save costs, but are not as easy to display. Pamphlets average about fifty cents to four dollars each and need to be regularly replenished. Conscientious data collection pays off. Staff don't want to overstock and end up with too many pamphlets in storage, nor order too few and have gaps on the shelf. There are no pamphlet fulfillment agencies, but vendors often allow bulk orders for a single title. A package of fifty brochures may cost ten dollars.

Some database vendors now offer eBrochures as part of their subscriptions or as standalone products. Databases typically start at one thousand dollars annually and may be priced based on patient beds, full-time employees, or library users. These products can carry thousands of titles and are updated in a timely fashion.

Free printed pamphlets are still available. The Consumer and Patient Health Information Section of the Medical Library Association publishes *Sources for Free Consumer Health Materials* (http://caphis.mlanet.org/chis/freeconsumer.html). Local public health agencies and community groups often partner with libraries to perform outreach to special populations by providing brochures. For example, the Houston Academy of Medicine-Texas Medical Center Library worked with community partner funding to translate and place health brochures in Asian temples and an Asian grocery store (Halsted, Varman, Sullivan, and Nguyen, 2002).

Technologies

Consumer health materials are available in multimedia formats, including DVD, CD-ROM, digitized books, etc. Consumer health films or educational CD-ROM programs can cost ten to three hundred dollars per title. The Consumer and Patient Health Information Section of the Medical Library Association *Sources for Free Consumer Health Materials* also contains multimedia materials.

Media programs need to be replaced if damaged, lost, or stolen. They also should be weeded or updated when new editions come out or the format becomes archaic, such as DVD replacing VHS format.

Multimedia naturally lends itself to an online environment. Networked televisions and computers can display films in continuous and on-demand systems in hospital waiting and recovery rooms. Services range from a single channel to an integrated system where films are stored on a server and played by request through a telephone, pillow-speaker, or computer. For integrated systems, the hardware, software, setup, licensing, and technical support is costly, starting at fifty thousand dollars and reaching hundreds of thousands of dollars per year. Other hospital departments, such as information systems, may help fund this service.

Bright Lights: There are many free consumer health films and animated tutorials online. The National Library of Medicine's MedlinePlus provides a Videos and Cool Tools section, with links to prescreened consumer health videos produced by hospitals, as well as their own National Institutes of Health Senior Health videos. Since the advent of YouTube and other self-production tools, healthcare providers can easily create and share films online for all to view or download.

Through online databases, patients and family members gain access to thousands of periodicals and books, along with powerful search interfaces. Starting at about one thousand dollars and upward to ten thousand dollars or more in annual licensing fees, databases are often out of reach of many consumer health libraries. Consortia members may be able to purchase databases cooperatively at discount.

Online Public Access Catalogs (OPACs), and more recently Discovery Tools, let library users search for resources within the collection, and usually cost two thousand dollars and up annually. Consortia may purchase an OPAC for all their members with shared savings. While it is possible for libraries to create their own OPACs and Discovery Tools using free open source software, the level of technical knowledge required is steep.

Kiosk terminals allow twenty-four/seven self-service access to consumer health resources. The Tampa General Hospital Foundation received a private grant of twenty thousand dollars for its Patient Education Resource Center, which included a freestanding kiosk with computer cubicles on both ends and space for one hundred pamphlets in the hospital's main lobby. The annual budget needed for toner, paper, and staff (volunteers ordered toner) was less than two hundred dollars (Northrop, Meehan, and Hatfield, 2012).

There are electronic tools available for purchase to simplify all aspects of library management: serials, acquisition, interlibrary loans, etc. These are often sold by subscription or OPAC vendors as part of an Integrated Online Library System, or they may be standalone products. Costs range from one thousand to tens of thousands of dollars annually.

Office Supplies

A consumer health information service uses similar supplies as do most offices—paper, staples, paper clips, etc. A library may be considered part of another department and ordering may be done centrally. About $125 a month is a practical estimate for office supplies. Printer cartridges alone usually cost forty-five to one hundred dollars.

Savings are possible through savvy management and thrift. Mailing enve-
lopes can be reused. Buying generic or recycled supplies and buying in bulk or
during sales saves costs. Paper clips will probably never become outdated, and
if there is space to store five thousand, there may be enough for a long time.
Organizations or consortia prefer vendors that sell supplies at discounted
rates. Some consortia also have email lists of giveaway supplies, and may offer
items no longer of use to other libraries for free.

Libraries often require materials that office supply stores do not carry,
such as book spine labels and pockets, brochure holders, etc. These can be
ordered through library supply vendors or purchased at discount in larger
quantities through consortia. In general, library supplies are not costly; a
roll of one thousand spine label protectors only costs about forty dollars
and should last for years.

Miscellaneous Costs

Depending on what services a resource center offers, there may be other
costs that do not fall into standard categories. Table 4.3 estimates costs of
common miscellaneous items and services.

TABLE 4.3
Cost Estimates of Miscellaneous Consumer Health Supplies and Services

Type of supply or service	Estimated cost in 2013
Binding and preservation	$10.00 and up per title
Bookmobile or outreach van	$25,000 and up, plus gas, insurance, taxes
Catering and food platters	$25.00 and up
Classes, conferences, registration, travel, etc.	$25.00–$500.00 per class or conference
Consultants	$50.00 per hour and up
Health fair materials	posters $4.00 and up, giveaways $1.00 and up
Interlibrary loan/document delivery	$5.00–$25.00 each, free if in FreeShare
Logo design	$100 and up
Photocopying	$0.05–$0.15 per page
Postage and shipping	$3.00 and up to mail an average book
Printing (brochures, bookmarks, pens, etc.)	$1.00 and up each, cost savings for bulk orders
Professional association memberships	$25.00–$300.00 each
Speaker fees and stipends for instructors	$25.00 and up
Travel expenses*	$0.565 per mile traveled in privately owned car
Website design	$50.00 per hour and up
Website hosting	Free to costs between $4.00–$1,000 per month

*For federal mileage reimbursement rates, see http://www.gsa.gov/portal/category/104715.

Facilities and Furniture

Visitors to consumer health information centers will need carpets to walk on, chairs to sit on, tables to read on, lighting to read by, and shelves and display racks to view resources on. Each computer needs a table or workstation and a chair. Each staff person needs a workspace with a desk and chair. At minimum, a patient family resource room should provide a table for four visitors with comfortable chairs, a computer workstation with a task chair, and a shelving unit with at least four shelves to display materials. A conservative estimate for these materials would be four thousand dollars, but many resource rooms will need a great deal more than these basic furnishings to meet their service goals.

Consortia sometimes list furnishings no longer needed, provided that someone can pick them up from the offering library.

When a new center is established, costs of construction and furniture are built into the initial proposal and budget. The center's manager often works with a planning committee, board, architects, contractors, interior designers, vendors, and staff to purchase everything from door signs to the color of paint for the walls. There may be multiple rooms, including bathrooms, kitchenettes, and classrooms that need to be built and furnished.

Furniture is usually considered a capital expenditure, and managers may need special permission from the parent organization for replacement. Sometimes furniture is ordered centrally through a facilities department. Organizations may have standards for vendors, colors, and materials, or restrictions due to fire codes.

If the consumer health information service manager is able to select furniture, ordering can be done through library and/or office supply vendors. Delivery and installation costs are usually extra. Because libraries are high-traffic areas and their furniture is made with care for durability and frequent use, it is not surprising for individual pieces to cost over three thousand dollars. While a substantial initial investment, most furniture lasts for at least ten years.

Equipment

Computers, printers, handheld devices, telephones, fax machines, photocopiers, scanners, televisions, CCTVs, digitized book players, and other technologies are integral parts of today's consumer health information services. Patient education television services require special television sets, and sometimes a server and bedside control devices. Cost of equipment is usually built into the initial center proposal and budget. Most businesses have an information systems department or consultant, who can work with the center's manager and planners on what equipment is needed.

Equipment may be considered a capital expenditure and ordered centrally. There may be specific standards or models, as networked equipment needs to be compatible throughout a site.

Each computer purchased will need at minimum a hard drive, monitor, keyboard, mouse, cables, and surge protector. The estimated cost for a basic computer is $1,200, a laptop $1,500, a computer on wheels for laptops approximately $2,500, and a desktop computer on wheels approximately $3,000 to $6,000. Printers vary based on model, functions, and features, and one printer can service multiple computers.

High-speed Internet connections are essential; costs will vary and may need to be budgeted separately, especially if the library is physically separated or not linked to the hospital network.

Bright Lights: Cost savings can be realized by bundling products; many modern photocopiers do double or even quadruple duty by also serving as printers, faxes, and scanners. Used equipment may be offered free through consortia lists, but usually require pick up and do not include installation or maintenance.

Ongoing costs include service and repairs, unless that is handled centrally by the information systems department. Annual or multiyear service contracts may be more cost-effective than one hundred to three hundred dollars per hour for onsite technicians every time equipment needs repairs.

Technology generally needs to be replaced or upgraded every three to ten years.

Personnel

Usually the largest part of the budget, personnel costs include salaries and benefits. The resource center manager may oversee the personnel budget, or budgeting may be done through a department or centrally for the organization or region. Full-time staff (often exempt and paid by annual salary) may be budgeted differently from part-time, nonexempt, hourly rate, or per-diem staff. Another differentiation commonly used is professional staff (with a master's of library science or equivalent degree) and paraprofessional (without the degree). Some organizations may use a step or grade program and set salaries based on skills needed for a job and years of service in that position. There will be a minimum and a maximum salary someone can make in a job in a step model.

Consumer health information services can be staffed by a solo practitioner, staff, and/or use temporary personnel to fill gaps. In addition to library science professionals and paraprofessionals, centers may be staffed by nurses, health educators, patient education specialists, and others. For example, an organization may hire a board-certified lactation consultant to teach a patient education class or support one of their nurses to become certified; the exam ranges from $460 to $640 (Howell, James, and Parsons, 2012). Staff can be paid through the operational budget or through grants or special purpose funds.

Most organizations have human resource departments or specialists to help managers understand the personnel budget. Professional association surveys, such as the Medical Library Association and Special Library Association salary surveys, can help develop appropriate salaries. The U.S. Bureau of Labor Statistics *Occupational Outlook Handbook* is a credible data source. The handbook lists $54,500 as the median U.S. librarian salary in 2010, $26,330 for library assistants and technicians, and $45,830 for health educators (U.S. Department of Labor, 2013). The range of salaries for library positions is highly variable and depends on factors such as organization size, geographic region, urban or rural community, university or government affiliation, and numerous other circumstances.

Employee performance is usually reviewed annually, and staff may receive merit salary increases of 1 to 5 percent a year. Some organizations allow bonuses, such as a holiday bonus of five hundred dollars, to all staff or to star performers.

Employee benefits can include, but are not limited to, health, dental, vision, prescription drug, short-/long-term care, life, and disability insurance for staff and their families/partners, vacation, holiday and sick time, family medical leave, child and dependent care, transportation and parking, and wellness programs. The consumer health resource center manager is not expected to select benefits for staff; the human resources or benefits department typically handles this function. For centers that are part of government agencies, benefits may be mandated. Additionally, staff may select insurance products among those offered, or opt out from receiving benefits. Given this, it is often difficult for a resource center manager to develop a first year personnel budget without historical data.

Sources of Funding

This chapter has focused on the expense side of the equation. Obviously, expenses need to be funded for the consumer health information service to open and run. In an ideal world, administrators could guarantee generous salaries, benefits and raises, top-of-the-line furniture, resources to meet every need, and extra funding for a bounty of special programs. In reality, consumer health resource centers are often underfunded, subject to cutbacks, or completely reliant on gifts and donations. It was estimated that during the "Great Recession" of 2009, most libraries endured some type of budget reductions, some as much as 40 percent (Bandy and Dudden, 2011). In the worst case scenario, salary is only provided for one part-time manager, but no funding for resources, because an administrator erroneously believes, "you can get everything online nowadays."

Fortunately, consumer health information managers are smart and savvy, and can often find ways to supplement minimal budgets through grants, donations, and grassroots fundraising.

Funding a New Service

Building a new consumer health information service from the ground up requires more money than organizations usually have on hand for everyday operations. The Massachusetts General Hospital Development Office actively sought a donor to secure adequate funds to build and staff the Patient Family Learning Center and provide ongoing funds for program development, educational materials, and equipment (Pittman, O'Connor, Millar, and Erickson, 2001). The Health Science Center at the University of Florida (affiliated with Shands Teaching Hospital) developed strategies to link the academic library with a local public library to provide services for patients and families. Stakeholders included the State Library of Florida, Bureau of Interlibrary Cooperation, and the Florida Library Network. The Patient Health Information Delivery System was funded through a grant (Coggan, 1993). Raising funds for a new center can take well over a year and is sometimes completed before the center's manager is hired.

Grants and Awards

Grants are available from many sources, including foundations, local businesses, civic groups, religious and fraternal organizations, and professional associations. Public libraries can apply for government funding through the State Aid to Public Libraries program. State boards of library commissioners provide funding to all types of libraries; for example, the Massachusetts General Hospital Treadwell Library was the site of the Consumer Health Reference Center funded by the Massachusetts Board of Library Commissioners (Stone, 2004). The Medical Library Association offers grants, such as the Librarians without Borders' Grant and the Research, Development, and Demonstration Project Grant. The National Library of Medicine also provides grants through its national and regional offices, including research grants, awards supporting career development and training, and support for outreach initiatives to improve access and eliminate health disparities. St. John's Hospital developed the Consumer Health Education and Promotion Project, funded partially by an impact grant from the National Network of Libraries of Medicine-Mid-Continental Region. The grant provided funding for travel expenses, presentation equipment, and temporary staff and enabled 390 visits to health clinics, public libraries, and county health departments (Morgan, Crabtree, and Henderson, 2006).

The Institute of Museum and Library Services is another source for grants, including projects related to literacy and those serving culturally diverse groups such as the elderly and people with disabilities.

Restricted grants are grants that must be used for a specific purpose (such as collecting materials in a certain language); unrestricted grants may be spent in any way the manager deems appropriate. Grantees must report at regular periods how the grants are being applied and complete a final report for the grantor.

Grant application is an involved and lengthy process, and requires excellent writing and organizational skills. It is a learned competence, and it's beneficial to take a class, read a book, or work with an expert before starting out. There are many reference books and online sources that list grant sources, such as *The Foundation Directory*. Larger organizations have grants departments to facilitate the process, and many grantors offer assistance or post instructions online. The Consumer and Patient Health Information Section of the Medical Library Association provides grant-writing tips for consumer health projects (http://caphis.mlanet.org/chis/grantwriting.html). Once a grant is awarded, a section of the budget is established where the money can be accessed until the end of the grant period.

Special purpose funds are restricted gifts established to serve distinct functions. They can come from an endowment, foundation, will, bequest, legacy, trust, estate, or internal or external donors. The Brigham and Women's Hospital Kessler Health Education Library benefited from a special purpose fund established by the family of a former orthopedic surgeon to provide orthopedic education; the fund provided books, brochures, and anatomical teaching models. Special purpose funds may be invested to generate additional income, similar to a bond fund.

Individuals and groups may wish to make donations, either as physical resources (books, artwork, furniture, etc.), money, or time (volunteering). A policy should outline what the center will accept and what will be done with donations not accepted. Monetary donations are usually welcome, unless they are restricted to a program the consumer health information service is not able to implement. Resources are welcome if they meet the library's collection development criteria, and are not damaged or moldy. Wish lists can be disseminated to potential donors to request what the library truly needs. Donations of volunteer time should be managed through the human resources, personnel, or volunteer department. For all donations, whether accepted or not, a note of appreciation should be sent to the giver. Donors can also be thanked through bookplates and invitations to the center.

Other methods of financing consumer health information services include loans, bonds, and leasing options. Managers pursuing these options should work with the organization's finance department.

Generating Revenue

Consumer health information service managers should contact appropriate departments before embarking on fundraising, such as finance, accounting, compliance, legal, boards, friends groups, etc., to determine whether and how funds can be collected and applied, especially for nonprofit organizations. Friends and auxiliary volunteers probably have more time than the manager to actively fundraise. Libraries themselves can generate income through interlibrary loans (five to twenty-five dollars), overdue fees (five to twenty-five cents), photocopying (five to fifteen cents), book sales (twenty-five cents and up), classes (twenty-five to two hundred dollars), consulting (fifty dollars and up), royalties for staff-authored books, and even bake sales. The Michigan Comprehensive Health Educational System staff offset some of their newsletter printing costs by selling advertisements to on-staff physicians. They also recommended developing reimbursable community educational offerings, such as diabetes education programs, that meet reimbursement criteria for planning, content, hours of participation, and evaluation. It has been hypothesized that people may value a service more if a reasonable fee is charged (Coggan, 1993). Revenue can be deposited into the operational budget, a special purpose fund, or used as petty cash.

Budget Management Training and Support

Managers new to budgeting should be educated on basic accounting precepts. Like cataloging and classification, the world of finance and accounting has its own vocabulary, formulas, and acronyms.

Schools of library science incorporate budgeting into management courses, and many offer continuing education classes or let alumni audit classes. College courses in basic accounting may be helpful. Outside organizations and vendors may offer training sessions. Veteran managers who have effectively managed budgets can serve as mentors to those new to the role.

Ongoing Financial Management

The budget for the first two years of a consumer health information service will look vastly different from subsequent years. Vendors and software may change to align with ongoing needs. It will probably take time to gather enough data on utilization to determine which and how many resources are needed. It is important to keep records of all items purchased. Most organizations recommend retaining financial records for five to ten years.

Institutional budgets are usually reviewed annually, and managers are sometimes required to present statistics on usage and needs. "Agreeing on a budget is like all politics: negotiation, give-and-take, compromise, and respectful agreement/disagreement," states Anne M. Turner, author of *Managing Money: A Guide for Librarians* (Turner, 2007, p. 127). Even if the budget is increased, many costs will also rise. It is important to fund existing services and resources before planning new ones. Managers facing a flat or decreased budget should scrutinize statistics to find low-use items that may be dropped, and substitute free or lower cost alternatives.

Cost per use data can help managers decide which items to continue to fund. One view of an electronic title that costs one hundred dollars is one hundred dollars per use, but one hundred views of a five hundred dollar title is only five dollars per use, so the second has a better cost per use ratio.

Managers should review budget reports regularly. In theory, one-twelfth of the budget should be expended each month, but costs are not typically distributed evenly over the year. A variance in one month may reflect a one-time purchase or seasonal fluctuation (Rykwalder, 1987). Unfamiliar charges in the monthly budget report should be brought to the budget or finance manager at the organization for an explanation and resolution if needed. Mistakes need to be addressed in a timely manner.

Financial management entails more than just tracking expenditures. Consumer health information service managers should create a financial plan that describes the program's anticipated accomplishments and what resources are necessary to achieve those goals (Bandy and Dudden, 2011). By and large, a budget is a critical tool for understanding and managing the resources and programs of a consumer health information service.

References

Bandy, M, and Dudden, RF. 2011. *The Medical Library Association Guide to Managing Health Care Libraries.* New York: Neal-Schuman.

Coggan, JM. 1993. "Funding a Patient Education Collection." *Bulletin of the Medical Library Association*, 81(4):435–37.

Halsted, DD, Varman, B, Sullivan, M, and Nguyen, L. 2002. "Consumer Health Information for Asians (CHIA): A Collaborative Project." *Journal of the Medical Library Association*, 90(4):400–405.

Howell, T, James, TF, and Parsons, L. 2012. "Building New Programs in Women's Health: A Fiscal Perspective." *International Journal of Childbirth Education*, (1):64+.

Morgan, A, Crabtree, B, and Henderson, HE. 2006. "Strengthening Consumer Health Information Delivery: An Education and Promotion Project." *Journal of Hospital Librarianship*, 6(3):1–17.

Northrop, L, Meehan, R, and Hatfield, B. 2012. "The Development and Implementation of a Freestanding Patient Education Resource Center (PERC)." *AAACN Viewpoint*, 34(1):3–5.

Pittman, TJ, O'Connor, MD, Millar, S, and Erickson, JI. 2001. "Patient Education: Designing a State-of-the-Art Consumer Health Information Library." *The Journal of Nursing Administration*, 31(6):316–23.

Reiners, LA. 2012. "Patron-driven Acquisition: The Experience of Three University Libraries." *SCONUL* Focus, 55(8):33–37.

Rykwalder, A. 1987. "Achieving Fiscal Fitness: Budgeting Basics for Patient Education Managers." *Patient Education and Counseling*, 9(1):73–79.

Stone, ME. 2004. "Librarian-to-Librarian: The Consumer Health Reference Center (CHRC) Experience." *Journal of Consumer Health on the Internet,* 8(1):1–11.

Turner, AM. 2007. *Managing Money: A Guide for Librarians.* Jefferson, NC: McFarland & Co.

U.S. Department of Labor. 2013. *Occupational Outlook Handbook.* St. Paul, MN: Jist Works.

5

Consumer- and Patient-Friendly Technology: Today and Tomorrow

Gabe Rios and Emma O'Hagan

A CCORDING TO A 2013 PEW SURVEY, 72 percent of adults in the United States used the Internet to find health information in the past year while 35 percent used the Internet in an attempt to self-diagnose or to diagnose someone else (Fox and Duggan, 2013). Thirty-one percent of Americans surveyed had used their mobile phones to search for health information (Pew Internet and American Life Project, 2012). This same survey found that Latino and African American users were more likely to search for health information using their mobile phones, thus demonstrating the need for multiple platforms to facilitate quality health information access.

Despite broad adoption of the Internet and its popular use as a tool for finding health information, disparities in using it continue to exist. In yet another 2013 Pew report, 85 percent of American adults reported using the Internet. While 78 percent of high school graduates went online, Internet use was lower for individuals with less than a high school education—just 59 percent. In addition to low education, a lower income also affected Internet adoption, with 76 percent of households earning less than thirty thousand dollars per year using the web. Internet use is also lower among older Americans with only 56 percent of adults over age sixty-five online (Rainie, 2013). Consumer health librarians must take these factors into account when promoting health technology and online health resources. These tools require various levels of Internet access as well as a certain degree of health literacy, computer familiarity, and the ability to navigate the Internet (Ancker et al., 2011).

Computers and Health Literacy

The use of mobile or computer-based health tools requires three distinct types of literacy: health, information, and computer literacy. In a 2012 systematic review of health literacy test instruments, Collins and others (2012) sought ones that could be utilized in computer-based screening. Computer screening for health literacy is important as consumers find that health information is increasingly only available online. Healthcare providers may require patients to interact and communicate through technology (e.g., patient portals). It would be ideal if a health literacy assessment took place online, at the point of use, in order to more accurately and conveniently assess a patient's abilities. Two gold-standards instruments were identified, the Rapid Estimate of Adult Literacy in Medicine and the Test of Functional Health Literacy in Adults. The authors then identified studies that compared other health literacy instruments adapted for use in computer-based environments to the gold standards.

In comparing these instruments to various other tests, the reviewers found the Health Literacy Screening Question Methodologies and the eHealth Literacy Scale displayed the most potential for computer-based screening. The authors caution that further testing of these instruments is needed to adequately adapt the tools to a reliable online or computer-based test (Collins et al., 2012).

Both the National Library of Medicine and the Office of Disease Prevention and Health Promotion provide recommendations for developing patient website information (U.S. Department of Health and Human Services and Prevention and Health Promotion, 2010). With these tips in mind, librarians evaluating and recommending patient-friendly websites should look for resources providing information at a sixth- or seventh-grade reading level. Literacy experts recommend a sixth-grade reading level as this ensures the information will be understandable to a large proportion of users. The organization of these materials is vital. To address literacy issues, shorter, segmented pieces focusing on a limited number of concepts are preferable to avoid overwhelming the reader. Consumer-level information should avoid abstract or vague statements and instead offer clear and executable instructions. Techniques that engage the reader, including stories or anecdotes and using the pronoun "you" in place of "the patient" are also recommended ("How to Write," 2013).

Patient-Friendly Web Resources

The websites provided by the National Institutes of Health, the National Library of Medicine, or the Agency for Healthcare Research and Quality

(AHRQ) serve as catalogs of high-quality consumer-level information. These websites aid librarians and healthcare providers in connecting consumer and patients to appropriate information. Among them are MedlinePlus (http://www.nlm.nih.gov/medlineplus/), TOXNET (http://toxnet.nlm.nih .gov/), ClinicalTrials.gov (http://clinicaltrials.gov/), AHRQ Patient Involvement: Diagnosis & Treatment (http://www.ahrq.gov/patients-consumers/ diagnosis-treatment/index.html), and National Institutes of Health Senior Health (http://nihseniorhealth.gov/).

Librarians should be aware of some information overlap among government-administered consumer health sites. For example, there are numerous, government-sponsored women's health sites including WomensHealth.gov, as well as women's health sites from the Centers for Disease Control and Prevention (http://www.cdc.gov/women/), the U.S. Food and Drug Administration (FDA; http://www.fda.gov/ForConsumers/byAudience/ForWomen/ default.htm), the National Institutes of Health (http://orwh.od.nih.gov/), and the National Library of Medicine (http://whr.nlm.nih.gov/). While each site may serve a different audience, each site may also link to or provide much of the same information. A patient might find it difficult to choose a source and may find the process of locating information as well as the redundancy of the information found fatiguing. Beginning with MedlinePlus, which links out to much of the same information and is a very comprehensive patient and consumer health resource, may help.

Bright Lights: It may be worth the effort to develop a catalog or index of useful and vetted, electronically available brochures. The University of Alabama at Birmingham's outpatient clinic, the Kirklin Clinic, has a small Patient Resource Library where librarians have developed an extensive index of brochures available to patients (http://www.uab.edu/lhluh/healthinfotopics). While valuable, developing such a resource can be time consuming and tedious. For many librarians, it may be preferable to rely on resources like MedlinePlus, a ready-made catalog for patient-friendly information.

Another type of consumer- and patient-friendly websites are symptom checkers. Symptom checkers cause anxiety among healthcare providers because consumers like to use them for self-diagnosis. These tools may sometimes provide accurate results; however, they can also be misleading or cause unnecessary worry—again because consumers may jump to conclusions (Ryan and Wilson, 2008; Usborne, 2009). Popular sites like WebMD (http://webmd.com) typically offer an exhaustive list of possible diseases or conditions, stating the most likely symptoms at the top. Once the symptoms are identified, a possible diagnosis results, although not in the context of the *likelihood* of the condition. The presence of pharmaceutical ads on these websites, often tied to symptoms the patient is researching, also raises important questions of intent on websites such as WebMD.

For consumers wanting symptom information, two more appropriate sites are Mayo Clinic's Symptom Checker (http://www.mayoclinic.com/health/symptom-checker/DS00671) and Symcat (http://symcat.com/). Mayo Clinic's symptom checker is smaller in scope than WebMD but offers more tempered information to consumers. Symcat (which stands for symptom-based, computer-assisted triage) is a relatively new site developed by two medical students from Johns Hopkins University. It calculates the likelihood of the user having a given condition based on prevalence. Possible diagnoses are drawn from data pulled from anonymous patient records from the Centers for Disease Control and Prevention (Walls, 2013). The site also directs patients to the type of healthcare provider most commonly consulted based upon an individual's symptoms. The creators of Symcat recognize most healthcare providers are wary of providing tools and information that can be used by a patient to evaluate symptoms. So, the purpose of Symcat is not to diagnose, but to offer an individual a reasonable consideration of his or her symptoms and then direct them to the appropriate medical provider. The developers used an algorithm with data from emergency departments and physicians' offices to calculate the likelihood that a symptom is one of a number of conditions or illnesses. The algorithm, a smart tool, will also learn from users as the site grows and, in turn, offer more accurate information ("Data-Driven Diagnosis," 2012).

HealthIT

These symptom-checker websites and many like them, while helpful to patients, are not consistently reviewed or regulated by federal law or oversight, which can promote quality, consistency, and ensure patients' and consumers' rights, such as their right to privacy of their personal health information. While not a regulatory body, the website HealthIT.gov includes a patient section that provides succinct descriptions of the types of technology available to promote patient care including electronic health records (EHRs). The site also discusses health information privacy and security, including what to do should a patient suspect his or her rights have been violated. A page devoted to finding and assessing quality health information resources provides patients with guidelines for evaluating online or mobile materials ("HeatlhIT.gov: Patients and Families," 2013.) Another government website, AHRQ.gov, devotes a segment of its site to providing very general information about diagnosis, healthcare planning, patient involvement, and prevention. These resources best serve patients in need of broad information as well as checklists and questions to prepare for an office visit or procedure, or to manage a change in their health status (Agency for Healthcare Research and Quality, 2013).

Another related federal initiative impacting consumer and patient technology is the Health Information Technology for Economic and Clinical Health (HITECH) Act signed into law in 2009, as part of the American Recovery and Reinvestment Act. The purpose of HITECH is to promote the adoption and meaningful use of health information technology for eligible healthcare professionals and hospitals. The Centers for Medicare & Medicaid Services developed the Eligible Professionals Decision Tool to determine eligibility for the Medicare and Medicaid EHR incentive programs (Centers for Medicare & Medicaid Services, 2013). There is a comparable tool to determine hospital eligibility on the cms.gov website. Eventually, healthcare professionals and hospitals will be required to meet "meaningful use" objectives to qualify for Medicare and Medicaid incentive payments. Stages 2 and 3 of this act will have a direct impact on two consumer- and patient-friendly technologies discussed here: personal health records (PHRs) and patient portals.

Personal Health Records

In 2003, the Markle Foundation funded a public-private collaborative working group to examine issues related to the PHR. The working group defines the PHR as: "an electronic application through which individuals can access, manage and share their health information, and that of others for whom they are authorized, in a private, secure, and confidential environment" (Connecting for Health Personal Health Working Group, 2003). PHRs function to empower consumers and ensure better continuity of care by providing a container to aggregate an individual's health-related documents. These documents could include:

- Advanced directives
- Allergy information
- Family history
- Health insurance information
- Health problems list
- Home monitored data

- Immunizations
- Laboratory tests
- List of procedures
- Major illnesses
- Medications
- Next of kin
- Provider list
- Social history and lifestyle

The documents are securely shared and privacy is protected to make sure healthcare providers have a full picture of their patient's health. Research on the potential benefits of PHRs suggests they help consumers be active participants in their healthcare by providing them the resources to be self-advocates and empowering them with readily accessible knowledge to ensure their continuity of care.

While there is much literature highlighting the hypothetical benefits of PHRs, there is little real-world evidence supporting their utility because their actual adoption rate remains very low. Pagliari and colleagues grouped potential benefits using the categories of patient empowerment, health gains, quality of care, and caregiver strain (Pagliari, Detmer, and Singleton, 2007). A significant patient empowerment benefit is the wide range of personal health information, data, and knowledge patients can leverage to improve their health and manage their disease(s). As a patient shares his or her PHR with various care providers, it becomes a preventive care tool by eliminating unnecessary tests and procedures and also helping care providers coordinate their care across medical disciplines, thus maximizing the potential for health gains. Improved quality of care results from more efficient provider-provider communication and provider-patient communication. The ability for providers to collaborate with each other on a patient's care plan is greatly increased if they have access to the same PHR with up-to-date information. More efficient provider-patient communication improves trust and treatment compliance. Lower costs, a decrease in unnecessary consultations, and reduced provider liability all serve to reduce the burden of care. These many benefits coupled with the convenience of having one place from which to retrieve personal health information make PHRs a key component to improved patient outcomes. So why isn't there a higher proliferation of them? According to a 2008 Markle Foundation public opinion survey on the potential and privacy considerations of electronic PHRs, "Americans overwhelmingly believe electronic personal health records could improve their health" (Connecting for Health, 2008). Approximately half of the public, 46.5 percent, are interested in using an online PHR service. Of those not interested, more than half cited concerns about privacy and confidentiality (Health Resources and Services Administration, 2013).

The overwhelming interest in PHRs coupled with pending federal requirements of the HITECH Act are an indication that there is a future for PHRs. National policies are needed to ensure that PHRs are interoperable with the network of EHR systems. Further blurring between PHRs and provider-administrated patient portals, discussed subsequently, will occur as data for these records becomes standardized and integrated.

Patient Portals

Patient portals are secure online tools that facilitate communication between patients and their healthcare providers (Health Resources and Services Administration, 2013). Though most frequently used to facilitate communication between provider and patient, portals are also important for patient self-management, particularly among patients with chronic illnesses or those who are unable to easily access a clinic. This is complicated by the fact that patients with multiple chronic health conditions are less likely to have Internet access (Fox and Purcell, 2010), thereby precluding their ability to use a patient portal for disease self-management.

Other features frequently available through patient portals include prescription refill requests, appointment scheduling, access to personal health records, bill payment features, and health education materials. This last component has the greatest implications for consumer health librarians. Resources commonly used by consumer health librarians when serving patients can be integrated into patient portals to promote quality health information, tailored to a patient's needs. MedlinePlus has developed a system to provide consumer-level information through patient portals (MedlinePlus Connect, 2012).

There is little evidence in the literature that many health science or hospital libraries are well integrated into patient portal systems, despite the opportunity for direct delivery of patient-specific, quality consumer health resources through a portal. Perhaps this is a result of the complications of implementing EHRs with patient portal components.

A 2009 study identified features of Kaiser Permanente PHR that increased use among consumers. They found that traffic increased if features patients perceived useful were available, regardless of ease of use (Silvestre, Sue, and Allen, 2009). The most useful components for the patients were communication features with healthcare providers, scheduling and bill payment, the ability to view their medical records, and access to health information (Eng and Lee, 2013). Healthcare providers and consumer health librarians are

Bright Lights: Vanderbilt University is an exception where librarians from the Eskind Biomedical Library have provided quality consumer-level information to patients through the MyHealthAtVanderbilt (MHAV) Portal. Librarians and information specialists at Vanderbilt were already well positioned to provide patient information through the patient portal thanks to their Patient Informatics Consult Service. This service allowed patients to request information through a Prescription for Information. When MHAV was redeveloped in 2005, the Prescription for Information service was shifted to the online patient portal platform, allowing librarians to potentially serve a greater number of patients by offering topical health and laboratory tests information and health news stories via the MHAV (Koonce, Giuse, Beuregard, and Giuse, 2007).

encouraged to advocate for the inclusion of health information on patient portals. As the platforms improve, expect new capabilities to improve ease of use, particularly features that assist patients in self-management and monitoring, perhaps through medical apps that integrate within EHRs and their corresponding patient portals (Eng and Leem 2013).

mHealth

An emerging trend to assist patients in self-management and monitoring is mHealth. mHealth can be defined as "medical and public health practice supported by mobile devices, such as mobile phones, patient monitoring devices, tablets, personal digital assistants (PDAs), and other wireless devices" (mHealth Alliance, 2013a). In general, mHealth is akin to personalized medicine or personalized health. It takes the right information along with access to service providers and puts them into the pocket of the patient. Using mHealth, providers can give patients basic information or they can engage in more advanced care like telehealth or teleradiology. Despite the lack of evidence, mHealth has the potential to foster disease prevention and lower readmission costs.

One of the biggest challenges facing mHealth is building evidence for positive outcomes. The University of Maryland completed a Mobile Diabetes Intervention Study to determine whether patient participation in decision-making about diabetes care is associated with better understanding of diabetes self-management and subsequent self-care practices (Quinn et al., 2009). Through automatic text messages, feedback, and coaching from healthcare providers, the study concluded that participation in decision-making plays a key role in patient understanding of diabetes self-management and subsequent self-care practices. This example of mHealth proved to be effective in facilitating behavior change and improving the connection between the patient and the provider (Smith, 2013).

As technology and interest in mHealth have matured in the last five years, an international collaboration called the mHealth Alliance developed to maximize the impact of mobile health by focusing on interoperability and open standards. The strategic priorities of the mHealth Alliance highlight five areas that hinder mHealth from becoming part of mainstreamed health systems. The five areas include evidence of benefit, technology interoperability, financing, global and national policies, and the community with capacity. Studies with high levels of evidence are needed for mHealth to have any potential to move towards mainstream adoption within health systems. As evidence is augmented, companies developing mHealth products and services will need to move towards open standards and interoperability to increase adoption. Promoting financing of mHealth initiatives will inspire innovation in the mHealth field. There is also potential cost-saving benefits as mHealth is adopted, especially in underserved markets. Global and national policies will help with mainstream adoption and ensure open standards. The mHealth Alliance seeks to build a community with capacity to support and build mHealth products and services that will have a broad benefit across different populations (mHealth Alliance, 2013b).

There are some remarkable examples of the capabilities of mHealth that support the strategic priorities of the mHealth Alliance. In a February 2012 TedTalk, Myshkin Ingawale, the co-founder of the med tech company Biosense Technologies, mentions the development of an mHealth device/app that will "democratize healthcare." The device, called "ToucHb," performs blood testing of hemoglobin without needles using an optical principle and light. The device also measures blood oxygen levels and heart rate. The device was developed for accredited social health activists in India with the intention of decreasing anemia-related deaths. ToucHb is simple to use, requires no needles, and is small enough for an accredited social health activist worker to carry in a kit. Accredited social health activist workers can diagnose anemia at the point of care and use a mobile app to send the test results anywhere (Ingawale, 2012). Biosense Technologies also develops a patient empowerment app with cost-savings potential due to disease prevention. "Uchek" performs a urine analysis to reveal potential health issues in an individual's urine. The app requires a smartphone and commercially available test strips. Using the built-in camera, consumers take a couple of photos of the strip at specified intervals over a few minutes. Using a similar technology to apps that read barcodes or QR codes, the app will read the color of those strips and provide information regarding the chemical composition of the urine and interpret what it means (Taylor, 2013).

mHealth has great potential to improve the overall health of an individual given the 2013 Pew Smartphone Ownership report that states 56 percent of adults own a smartphone (Smith, 2013). The real value for mHealth is using the data collected with apps and devices to improve patient or consumer engagement in their own health.

Quantified Self

Self-tracking and using health data are part of a new movement called "Quantified Self" (QS). This movement creates new opportunities to promote consumer engagement in health and wellness. There is no generally accepted definition of QS; however, Wikipedia states "QS is a movement to incorporate technology into data acquisition on aspects of a person's daily life in terms of inputs (e.g., food consumed, quality of surrounding air), states (e.g., mood, arousal, blood oxygen levels), and performance (mental and physical)" ("Quantified Self," 2013). The most concise definition can be found at quantifiedself.com, which has the tagline of "self knowledge through numbers" (Quantified Self Labs, 2013).

The QS movement has gained prominence due to the number of consumer- and patient-friendly technologies readily available. These technologies track steps taken, sleep patterns, or calories burned. The QS tracking devices available are somewhat comparable so, in addition to reviewing standard features, differences in the most popular activity tracking devices (Fitbit [http://www.fitbit.com/], Body Media [http://www.bodymedia .com/], Jawbone [http://www.jawbone.com], and Nike+™ FuelBand [http:// www.nike.com/us/en_us/c/nikeplus-fuelband]) are highlighted here. All of these devices track the number of steps taken and calories burned. In addition to these measurements, Fitbit, Body Media, and Jawbone track sleep patterns and sleep efficiency. Each tracking device offers a suite of complementary web applications or mobile apps that allow the user to upload data from their device. Additionally, some devices have a built-in display. The Fitbit One can display steps taken, distance traveled, calories burned, and floors climbed. The Fitbit One also displays a flower that grows and shrinks based upon an individual's recent activity. The Body Media family of armband devices does not have a built-in display, but there is an optional display device that wirelessly communicates with the armband to show calories burned, steps taken, and activity as it happens. The display also alerts the user when daily targets are met and features comparable armband data from today and yesterday. The Nike+™ FuelBand has a minimal display that tracks steps taken and calories burned.

Some device makers offer specialized services (for example, Lark [http://lark.com/], a sleep tacking device that helps people understand and enhance their sleep quality through monitoring and online counseling. This device is unique from the other devices previously mentioned that track sleep patterns because it features a wristband that wakes the user silently and gently with vibration. More recently, Lark released the Lark Life, which is comparable to the Fitbit family of devices feature-wise.

One of the latest entrants into this market is the Basis B1 Band (http://www.mybasis.com/). Distinctive features of this device are measurement of optical blood flow (heart rate data) and "gamification," the use of game thinking and game mechanics to engage individuals in healthy habits. The devices range in price from sixty to two hundred dollars, with some requiring additional monthly fees to access a web dashboard interface providing data and counseling.

In addition to these tracking devices, there are several activity-tracking and food diary apps for smartphones. For example, activity-tracking running apps include the popular Runkeeper (http://runkeeper.com/) and Map My Run (http://www.mapmyrun.com/). Both are mature apps and provide distance, calories burned, maps using a smartphone's GPS, social features, and goal setting. The social features of the running apps allow individuals to motivate friends and share running routes. The goal-setting features act like a personal trainer by setting up a training plan to run anything from a 5K to a marathon. Moves (http://www.moves-app.com/), similar to the running apps, tracks additional activities such as walking and cycling, using the smartphone's ability to measure movements (e.g., accelerometer), and is less intrusive. The app runs in the background continuously and tracks everything the individual does, as long as the smartphone is present. The app displays the distance, duration, steps, and calories burned for each activity.

Keeping a food diary is a well-documented consumer approach to weight loss and wellness (Hollis et al., 2008). There are several apps to help consumers log their meals. Examples include Lose It (http://www.loseit.com/), Weight Watchers (http://www.weightwatchers.com/templates/Marketing/Marketing_Utool_1col.aspx?pageid=1118811), MyFitnessPal (http://www.myfitnesspal.com/), and LiveStrong MyPlate (http://www.livestrong.com/thedailyplate/). Most food diary apps have the same basic functionality, including a website interface to enter information in addition to a smartphone app. Research shows consumers have better adherence if they adopt an app on their smartphone (Acharya et al., 2011). In addition to the food diary, these apps offer goal-setting and social features similar to the activity-tracking apps. After inputting personal information, these apps ask the individual to set a goal weight, and a daily calorie budget is established. The food diary part of the apps allows individuals to track what they eat and drink by entering certain foods from a database or by using a built-in barcode scanner. Food is automatically recorded with the appropriate serving size, calories, and mac-ronutrients. If specific foods are not in the database, individuals can manually enter a food item or recipe and save it for future use. The food diary apps are more mature than some of the activity-tracking apps with data interoperabil-ity. Several of the food diary apps allow data from activity-tracking devices and apps to be imported into their web dashboards. Activity-tracking apps only recently started adding these features to their web dashboards.

More specialized apps focus on specific activities. In addition to the Lark sleep-tracking device noted previously, free or very low cost sleep-tracking apps with similar features include Sleep as Android (https://sites.google.com/site/sleepasandroid/), Sleep Cycle (http://www.sleepcycle.com/), and Sleep-Bot (http://mysleepbot.com/). Apps are also available to help patients keep up their medical records. VaxNation, for example, is an application that helps patients track their vaccinations (Walls, 2013).

While all these devices and apps help consumers establish healthy habits, there is room for improvement in the interoperability of data between these different devices and apps. More standardization is needed as the market continues to change and becomes saturated with similar devices and apps.

Health App Evaluation

Considering the vast number of health apps of sometimes dubious quality available to patients, consumer health librarians are often in a position to evaluate, recommend, or conversely steer patients away from them. Unfor-tunately, there are few resources to help consumer health librarians, let alone patients and healthcare providers, sift through the glut of health apps. In the spring and summer of 2012, many estimates suggested there were more than forty thousand mobile health applications available (Pelletier, 2012; Walls, 2013). Only one year earlier, the *New York Times* reported that there were about seventeen thousand health apps (Koleskikov-Jessop, 2011). An October 2012 issue of the *Association of American Medical Colleges Reporter* cited a report by Juniper Research that predicted 44 million downloads of health ap-plications for 2012 and a predicted increase to 142 million downloads in 2016 (Pelletier, 2012). Clearly, the number of health apps is challenging to health professionals and consumers alike.

That said, a few organizations are working to aid providers and consum-ers in discovering and assessing apps for meaningful use. Johns Hopkins University's Global mHealth Initiative promotes and carries out studies to evaluate the impact of mobile health interventions. Some randomized controlled trials and clinical reviews are also beginning to appear in medical journals (Pelletier, 2012).

According to a 2012 report from *MobiHealthNews*, the most commonly available consumer medical apps largely support general wellness through diet, exercise, and stress management. Other major categories include medication adherence and managing chronic conditions (Dolan, 2012). A limited number of research trials have been published evaluating medical applications, and fewer still concentrate on the kind of patient-focused applications widely adopted. User-posted reviews may be the only source of appraisal for some apps. Blogs of varying quality are a popular and current source of app evaluation. The *iMedical App Blog*, produced by a team of physicians, medical students, and other allied health professionals, is an excellent resource for reviews of many popular medical apps. The blog also serves as a resource for discovering new applications. Should a reader discover an app that has not been reviewed on *iMedical App Blog*, there is a "submit an app review" feature (http://www.imedicalapps.com/). The Cochrane Collaboration lists the *iMedical Apps Blog* among their list of evidence-based healthcare resources (The Cochrane Collaboration, 2013).

MobiHealthNews blogger Brian Dolan has written extensively about the need for curation of mobile health applications (*MobiHealthNews*, 2013). Because there are few authoritative sources for evaluating medical applications, a resource helping patients and providers identify high quality health, wellness, and fitness apps is sorely needed. The DocGuide Apps site (http://dgapps.docguide.com/) evaluates apps for healthcare providers and categorizes them by specialty. Unfortunately, it does not include applications specifically designed for patients. One resource to watch is Happtique, a subsidiary of Greater New York Hospital Association Ventures. Until recently, Happtique largely focused on creating a single-purpose health app store to serve hospitals and other healthcare organizations. It's now developing a voluntary Health App Certification Program to "help healthcare practitioners, patients, and consumers identify clinically and technically sound apps from among the 40,000-plus health, medical, and fitness apps in iTunes, Google Play, and other public app stores" ("Happtique Launches mRx," 2012). In its proposed certification standards, mobile health apps must meet operability, privacy, security, and content requirements for certification (Happtique Inc., 2013). Check their website for progress on this promising program (http://www.happtique.com/).

Both organizations and industry publications have created lists of mobile health applications but often skirt the quality issue by refusing to endorse the resources, thereby doing little to guide users to reliable tools. HealthIT.gov publishes one such list of "wellness apps," which includes popular resources like Lose It!, My Fitness Pal, and Healthy Cloud, but the list stops short of endorsing a specific product and is too brief to offer users more than a surface idea of what is available ("HealthIT.gov: Stay Well," 2013). *MobiHealthNews*, for example, has published a report that examines trends among over thirteen thousand consumer health apps available for iOS devices ("An Analysis of Consumer Health Apps," 2012). These types of resources can guide health-care executives but do little to inform the average consumer.

Literature to Discover and Evaluate Mobile Health Apps

As previously mentioned, there are few studies discussing the proven out-comes and the effectiveness of mobile health applications. Consumers and healthcare providers alike are in need of resources to help identify appropri-ate, high-quality applications. Slowly, studies examining the quality of mobile health tools are being published. A number of systematic reviews have ap-peared, some of which examine mobile health applications in general or those specifically designed for consumers. In a 2012 systematic review, Mosa, Yoo, and Sheets divided mobile health applications into three categories: health-care professionals, health science students, and patients. The review identified only fourteen studies discussing fifteen patient-level applications (Mosa, Yoo, and Sheets, 2012). The findings suggest that more research is needed to evalu-ate consumer health mobile tools.

A 2013 systematic review examined seventy-five controlled trials of applica-tions and other mobile-based interventions for healthcare consumers. Accord-ing to the review, most of the identified studies were of low quality, further proving that the need for more rigorous evaluative studies of mobile health-care technology (Free et al., 2013). This same review suggests there is mixed evidence for the efficacy of consumer health, mobile technology interventions, again underscoring the need for better quality studies along with improvements to the interventions and technologies currently in use (Free et al., 2013).

Although a few studies have attempted to review mobile health applica-tions, many stop short of assessing quality. This may be a result of the rapid growth of the mobile health app market. The job of evaluating mobile health applications, even when focusing on a relatively limited subset of health apps such as those specific to endocrine disorders, is simply too large and difficult. For example, in a 2013 review of diabetes and endocrinology apps, a search of the iPhone App Store yielded six hundred applications. The number of life-style, nutrition, and other general wellness apps seems to be especially over-whelming to medical researchers (Eng and Lee, 2013). Librarians interested in mobile health can also follow the *Journal of Mobile Technology in Medicine*, a new peer-reviewed, open access journal first published in 2012.

mHealth and Chronic Disease Management

One of the most exciting opportunities mobile technology provides is in chronic disease management. Applications and online tools are available for patients with diabetes (El-Gayar, Timsina, Nawar, and Eid, 2013; Eng and Lee, 2013), congenital heart disease (Klausen et al., 2012), and asthma and allergies (Burnay et al., 2013), among others. These tools typically track a patient's health either through patient-entered logs or wearable devices. Typically, information is shared with a patient's healthcare provider and potentially integrated into the EHR. Ideally, educational materials are also pushed to the user through the mobile interface (Tsalatsanis et al., 2011). These tools may include social features for connecting patients with other individuals for additional support, suggest self-care modalities, or provide reminders about medication or other interventions. Because many of these specific mobile health applications store and transmit personal health information, there is a heightened need for regulation and monitoring. Recently, the Food and Drug Administration (FDA) began to address this need.

FDA Guidelines for Mobile Health Devices

In September 2013, the FDA published guidelines for the regulation of mobile medical applications. According to these guidelines, the FDA regulates anything that turns a mobile phone or tablet into a medical device as defined by the Food, Drug and Cosmetic Act (FD&C Act). By the FDA's definition, this would include applications where a mobile phone was used as an accessory to another medical device or any applications where the mobile phone or tablet became a medical device, including applications that read a patient's vital signs or makes diagnoses. Regulation is limited to applications and the FDA has no plans to regulate mobile device distributors or mobile app marketplaces like the iTunes Store or GooglePlay (U.S. Food and Drug Administration [FDA], 2013b).

Currently, developers of apps that qualify as medical devices are required to submit their apps to the FDA for evaluation under Section 501(K) of the FD&C Act (U.S. FDA, 2013a). However, the FDA's definition, noted above, does not include the vast majority of consumer health medical applications currently available. Prior to the release of these guidelines, the FDA released their classification system for software-based devices that store, transfer, or display medical data. Software and computer-based devices are classified as Class I, II, or III. Class I is considered low risk and is subject only to general controls like registration, adverse event reporting, and adequate design controls, while Class III is considered high risk and subject to premarket approval (U.S. FDA, 2013a; U.S. FDA, 2013b). This classification system determines the application's regulatory requirements.

The FDA does not regulate mobile apps that promote fitness or general wellness, including apps that track weight, posture, or calories. Because these apps are not intended to treat or diagnose, their use of accessories like scales, pedometers, or wearable devices are not regulated. Other examples of unregulated medical apps might include medical textbooks, reference resources, or point-of-care reference tools, including those used as teaching aids for patients. However, if the medical information app allows the patient or physician to input specific patient information to aid in diagnosis, the app falls under the FDA guidelines and is therefore subject to regulation. Under the guidelines, apps allowing users to access and view information in an EHR would not be regulated (U.S. FDA, 2013b).

Current FDA regulations have little effect on the availability of most patient apps while significantly impacting those used by or developed for clinicians. However, the absence of regulation or guidelines for apps marketed toward the consumer and not classified as mobile medical apps has implications for healthcare providers and consumer health librarians who evaluate and recommend these mobile tools to patients.

The Future

Consumer- and patient-friendly technology includes a broad array of apps, resources, services, and electronic devices; however, there are many issues impacting their widespread adoption, including their ease of use and ability to provide consumers and patients with actionable information. Several of these technologies prove that health behavior can be modified through continued use. Additionally, an important aspect of their use is the significant potential to connect patients to providers, expanding patient-provider communication. For a while, consumers and patients will see a blending of old and new models of healthcare delivery as these technologies continue to evolve, mature, and become accepted. Coupled with federal regulations such as HITECH, which stipulate requirements of more engaged patients, eHealth technologies have the capability to improve the quality of care while boosting patient satisfaction.

References

Acharya, SD, Elci, OU, Sereika, SM, Styn, MA, and Burke, LE. 2011. "Using a Personal Digital Assistant for Self-Monitoring Influences Diet Quality in Comparison to a Standard Paper Record among Overweight/Obese Adults." *Journal of the American Dietetic Association*, 111(4):583–88.

Agency for Healthcare Research and Quality. 2013. "Patients and Consumers." http://www.ahrq.gov/patients-consumers/index.html. Accessed June 10, 2013.

"An Analysis of Consumer Health Apps for Apple's iPhone 2012." 2012. *MobiHealthNews*, July 11, 2012. http://www.webcitation.org/69YHjptQ9. Accessed February 24, 2014.

Ancker, JS, Barron Y, Rockoff ML, Hauser D, Pichardo M, Szerencsy A, and Calman N. 2011. "Use of an Electronic Patient Portal among Disadvantaged Populations." *Journal of General Internal Medicine*, 26(10):1117–23.

Burnay E, Cruz-Correia R, Jacinto T, Sousa AS, and Fonseca J. 2013. "Challenges of a Mobile Application for Asthma and Allergic Rhinitis Patient Enablement-Interface and Synchronization." *Telemedicine Journal and E-Health*, 19(1):13–18.

Centers for Medicare & Medicaid Services. 2013. "EHR Incentive Programs." June 26, 2013. https://www.cms.gov/Regulations-and-Guidance/Legislation/EHRIncentive Programs/index.html?redirect=/ehrincentiveprograms/. Accessed February 28, 2014.

The Cochrane Collaboration. 2013. "Social Media Resources: Blogs." http://www.cochrane.org/about-us/evidence-based-health-care/webliography/social-media. Accessed February 28, 2014.

Collins, SA, Currie, LM, Bakken, S, Vawdrey, DK, and Stone, PW. 2012. "Health Literacy Screening Instruments for eHealth Applications: A Systematic Review." *Journal of Biomedical Informatics*, 45(3):598–607.

Connecting for Health. 2008. *Americans Overwhelmingly Believe Electronic Personal Health Records Could Improve Their Health*. Markel Foundation. June. http://www.markle.org/sites/default/files/ResearchBrief-200806.pdf. Accessed February 28, 2014.

Connecting for Health Personal Health Working Group. 2003. *The Personal Health Working Group: Final Report*. Markel Foundation. July 1, 2003. http://www.policy archive.org/collections/markle/index?section=5&id=15473. Accessed February 28, 2014.

"Data-Driven Diagnosis: A Google for Your Health Symptoms." 2012. *The Atlantic*. March 22, 2012. http://www.theatlantic.com/health/archive/2012/03/data-driven -diagnosis-a-google-for-your-health-symptoms/254506/. Accessed February 28, 2014.

Dolan, B. 2012. "New Trends for Consumer Health Apps." *MobiHealthNews*. July 24. http://mobihealthnews.com/17968/three-new-trends-for-consumer-health-apps/. Accessed February 28, 2014.

El-Gayar, O, Timsina, P, Nawar, N, and Eid, W. 2013. "Mobile Applications for Diabetes Self-Management: Status and Potential." *Journal of Diabetes Science and Technology*, 7(1):247–62.

Eng, DS, and Lee, JM. 2013. "The Promise and Peril of Mobile Health Applications for Diabetes and Endocrinology." *Pediatric Diabetes*, 14(4):231–38.

Fox, S, and Duggan, M. 2013. *Health Online 2013*. Pew Research Center. January 15, 2013. http://pewinternet.org/~/media//Files/Reports/PIP_HealthOnline.pdf. Accessed February 28, 2014.

Fox, S, and Purcell, K. 2010. *Chronic Disease and the Internet*. Pew Research Center. March 24, 2010. http://www.pewinternet.org/Reports/2010/Chronic-Disease.aspx. Accessed February 28, 2014.

Free, C, Phillips, G, Galli, L, Watson, L, Felix, L, Edwards, P, Patel, V, and Haines, A. 2013. "The Effectiveness of Mobile-Health Technology-Based Health Behaviour Change or Disease Management Interventions for Health Care Consumers: A Systematic Review." *PLoS Medicine*, 10(1):e1001362.

Happtique Inc. 2013. *Health App Certification Program: Certification Standards*. http://info.happtique.com/download-standards-post-form-submission?submission Guid=1a117bf1-7d9d-4ca0-a8ba-4e9745fc98a4. Accessed September 8, 2013.

"Happtique Launches mRx Pilot Program." 2012. *Skyline News*. August 27, 2012. http://www.gnyha.org/PressRoom/Publication/0c3f45faf80b4f2cb54cf851162ea e9e/. Accessed February 28, 2014.

"HeatlhIT.gov: Patients and Families." 2013. HealthIT.gov. http://www.healthit.gov/patients-families. Accessed June 1, 2013.

"HealthIT.gov: Stay Well." 2013. HealthIT.gov. http://www.healthit.gov/patients-families/stay-well. Accessed May 28, 2013.

Health Resources and Services Administration. 2013. "What Is a Patient Portal?" http://www.hrsa.gov/healthit/toolbox/HealthITAdoptiontoolbox/Personal HealthRecords/patientportal.html. Accessed June 10, 2013.

Hollis, JF, Gullion, CM, Stevens, VJ, Brantley, PJ, Appel, LJ, Ard, JD, Champagne, CM, et al. 2008. "Weight Loss during the Intensive Intervention Phase of the Weight-Loss Maintenance Trial." *American Journal of Preventive Medicine*, 35(2):118–26.

"How to Write Easy-to-Read Health Materials." 2013. National Library of Medicine. National Institutes of Health. http://www.nlm.nih.gov/medlineplus/etr.html. Accessed June 15, 2013.

Ingawale, M. 2012. "A Blood Test without Bleeding." TED video, 6:43. March 2012. http://www.medgadget.com/2012/03/myshkin-ingawale-a-blood-test-without -bleeding.html. Accessed February 28, 2014.

Klausen, SH, Mikkelsen, UR, Hirth, A, Wetterslev, J, Kjaergaard, H, Sondergaard, L, and Andersen, LL. 2012. "Design and Rationale for the PREVAIL Study: Effect of E-Health Individually Tailored Encouragements to Physical Exercise on Aerobic Fitness among Adolescents with Congenital Heart Disease—a Randomized Clinical Trial." *American Heart Journal*, 163(4):549–56.

Koleskikov-Jessop, S. 2011. "Do-It-Yourself Health Care with Smarthphones." *New York Times*. February 28, 2011. http://www.nytimes.com/2011/03/01/technology/01iht -srhealth01.html?pagewanted=all&_r=0. Accessed February 28, 2014.

Koonce, TY, Giuse, DA, Beauregard, JM, and Giuse, NB. 2007. "Toward a More Informed Patient: Bridging Health Care Information through an Interactive Communication Portal." *Journal of the Medical Library Association*, 95(1):77–81.

MedlinePlus Connect. 2012. "MedlinePlus Connect: Linking Patient Portals and EHRs to Consumer Health Information." US National Library of Medicine. http://www .nlm.nih.gov/medlineplus/connect/overview.html. Accessed February 28, 2014.

mHealth Alliance. 2013a. "MHealth Alliance: Frequently Asked Questions." http://www.mhealthalliance.org/about/faq. Accessed July 8, 2013.

mHealth Alliance. 2013b. "Strategic Priorities." http://www.mhealthalliance.org/our-work/strategy. Accessed February 28, 2014.

MobiHealthNews. 2013. "Home Page." http://mobihealthnews.com/. Accessed May 28, 2013.

Mosa, AS, Yoo, I, and Sheets, L. 2012. "A Systematic Review of Healthcare Applications for Smartphones." *BMC Medical Informatics and Decision Making,* 12:67.

Pagliari, C, Detmer, D, and Singleton, P. 2007. "Potential of Electronic Personal Health Records." *BMJ,* 335(7615):330–33.

Pelletier, SG. 2012. "Explosive Growth in Health Care Apps Raises Oversight Questions." *AAMC Reporter,* October. https://www.aamc.org/newsroom/reporter/october2012/308516/health-care-apps.html. Accessed February 28, 2014.

Pew Internet and American Life Project. 2012. *Mobile Health 2012.* Pew Research Center. November 8, 2012. http://www.pewinternet.org/Reports/2012/Mobile-Health.aspx. Accessed February 28, 2014.

"Quantified Self." July 21, 2013. *Wikipedia.* http://www.en.wikipedia.org/wiki/Quantified_Self. Accessed February 28, 2014.

Quantified Self Labs. 2013. "Quantified Self: Self Knowledge through Numbers." http://quantifiedself.com/. Accessed February 28, 2014.

Quinn, CC, Gruber-Baldini, AL, Shardell, M, Weed, K, Clough, SS, Peeples, M, et al. 2009. "Mobile Diabetes Intervention Study: Testing a Personalized Treatment/Behavioral Communication Intervention for Blood Glucose Control." *Contemporary Clinical Trials,* 30(4):334–46.

Rainie, L. 2013. *Internet Adoption Becomes Nearly Universal among Some Groups, but Others Lag Behind.* May 30, 2013. http://www.pewresearch.org/fact-tank/2013/05/30/internet-adoption-becomes-nearly-universal-among-some-groups-but-others-lag-behind/. Accessed February 28, 2014.

Ryan, A, and Wilson, S. 2008. "Internet Healthcare: Do Self-Diagnosis Sites Do More Harm than Good?" *Expert Opinion on Drug Safety,* 7(3):227–29.

Silvestre, AL, Sue, VM, and Allen, JY. 2009. "If You Build It, Will They Come? The Kaiser Permanente Model of Online Health Care." *Health Affairs (Project Hope),* 28(2):334–44.

Smith, A. 2013. *Smartphone Ownership 2013.* Pew Research Center. http://www.pewinternet.org/Reports/2013/Smartphone-Ownership-2013.aspx. Accessed February 28, 2014.

Taylor, C. 2013. "This App Will Test Your Pee." Mashable. February 25, 2013. http://mashable.com/2013/02/26/uchek-urine-analysis-app/. Accessed February 28, 2014.

Tsalatsanis, A, Gil-Herrera, E, Yalcin, A, Djulbegovic, B, and Barnes, L. 2011. "Designing Patient-Centric Applications for Chronic Disease Management." *Conference Proceedings: Annual International Conference of the IEEE Engineering in Medicine and Biology Society,* 2011:3146–49.

Usborne, S. 2009. "Cyberchondria: The Perils of Internet Self-Diagnosis." *The Independent.* February 17, 2009. http://www.independent.co.uk/life-style/health-and-families/features/cyberchondria-the-perils-of-internet-selfdiagnosis-1623649.html. Accessed February 28, 2014.

U.S. Department of Health and Human Services. Office of Disease, and Prevention and Health Promotion. 2010. *Health Literacy Online: A Guide to Writing and Designing Easy-to-Use Health Web Sites*. Washington, DC: U.S. Department of Health and Human Services. Office of Disease, and Prevention and Health Promotion. http://www.health.gov/healthliteracyonline/Web_Guide_Health_Lit_Online.pdf. Accessed February 28, 2014.

U.S. Food and Drug Administration. 2011. *Draft Guidance for Industry and Food and Drug Administration Staff Mobile Medical Applications*. http://www.fda.gov/downloads/MedicalDevices/DeviceRegulationandGuidance/GuidanceDocuments/UCM263366.pdf. Accessed February 28, 2014.

U.S. Food and Drug Administration. 2013a. "Medical Devices: 501K Clearances." http://www.fda.gov/medicaldevices/productsandmedicalprocedures/deviceapprovalsand clearances/510kclearances/default.htm. Accessed February 28, 2014.

U.S. Food and Drug Administration. 2013b. *Mobile Medical Applications: Guidance for Industry and Food and Drug Administration Staff*. September 25, 2013. http://www.fda.gov/downloads/MedicalDevices/.../UCM263366.pdf. Accessed March 24, 2014.

Walls, J. 2013. "Growing 'App'etite for Mobile Health." *Washington Post*. May 7, 2013. http://www.washingtonpost.com/sf/brand-connect/wp/2013/05/07/growing -appetite-for-mobile-health/. Accessed February 28, 2014.

6

Prized Assets: Staff

Jean Shipman and Erica Lake

"**I**F YOU'VE SEEN ONE CONSUMER LIBRARY, you have seen one consumer library." This could not be truer as far as staffing a consumer library. No two libraries will have the exact same needs. Staffing is influenced by location, hours of operation, library mission, and services. The one thing that is constant among consumer libraries is that staffing is the most important resource, and one that can either make or break a library's success.

Staff Composition

Staff composition may consist of any combination of full-time and part-time employees, salaried and hourly employees, librarians, library technicians and assistants, library aides, students, and volunteers. Every library will have its own unique staffing needs. This is especially true today, as consumer health librarians assume new responsibilities with electronic resources, virtual services, and information technology. Before staffing the library along traditional service lines, take time to assess what services and resources should or will be offered. Consider where the library will be located, its hours of operation, and the available budget.

Librarians

Librarians are the cornerstone of a consumer health library. Their professional library degrees and ongoing health information training have prepared them to expertly and efficiently serve patients, healthcare providers, and the general community. Consumer health libraries managed by a librarian with a professional library degree are the gold standard for staffing.

Non-Librarian Staff

Paraprofessional and nonprofessional staff are a vital presence in libraries. Though they do not have professional library degrees, they often receive training on the foundations of library service. Assigning complex library duties to paraprofessional and nonprofessional staff is fine as long as the librarian parameters of practice are clear to them. Provide these staff members with job competencies, formal mentoring, cross-training programs, career opportunity workshops, and continuing education classes to further their development.

Bright Lights: "A Case Study Based Training for Consumer Health Library Support Staff" is located on the Medical Library Association's Consumer and Patient Health Information Section website: http://caphis.mlanet.org/.

In any academic setting, there will be a plethora of students vying for library aide positions. The key to retaining them is to provide stimulating work and interesting tasks, along with a positive, productive work environment.

Bright Lights: Consider creating a library internship or practicum for students in health-related fields (e.g., public health or nursing) to expose them to patient education resources and means for effectively communicating with patients and their family members about these materials.

Though volunteers can be a valuable resource, there can be pros and cons to having them in the library. In lean times, supervisors may turn to volunteers in lieu of compensated staff as a quick fix to fill staffing vacancies, and then find they are dependent upon them to perform essential daily operations. Worse still in this scenario is the possible diminishment of the value of library professionals to organizational administrators, who may perceive the volunteer as performing just fine. Additionally, while retired healthcare professionals and health science alumni can be enthusiastic volunteers, they need to understand they may not practice healthcare in their role within the library. Conversely, utilizing volunteers can allow services to be expanded, and can free up librarians' time so they can engage in more professional tasks. Establishing a detailed volunteer program and remaining vigilant about maintaining salaried staff can help librarians avoid potential pitfalls associated with volunteer use.

Bright Lights: "Virtual volunteers" provide their donated services entirely over the Internet from a home computer and may be a good fit for some libraries. They can develop or update websites and blogs, look up articles, or write thank-you letters to donors. Virtual volunteers should be self-motivated, have good time management skills, and be both skilled and comfortable communicating in writing as email is the primary form of interaction.

Sources of Staff: What Kind of Librarian Is Best?

Where do librarians for a consumer library come from? Do they have to be medical librarians or have experience working in a health sciences library to be effective? Surprisingly, no. In fact, the skills and attributes of a public librarian are often a better match for a consumer library. Public librarians are used to developing programs that serve the information needs of the general community. Consumer health librarians frequently develop such programming and services. Public librarians are also accustomed to dealing with members of the general community, composed of individuals from all walks of life, cultural backgrounds, and health literacy levels. Trained public librarians work with diverse individuals to ascertain their true information needs.

Hospital librarians are another strong match as they have the ability to work with individuals from all facets of the hospital's patient population and may be adept at working independently. Like their public library counterparts, they are skilled at conducting a focused reference interview. Well versed in the types and capabilities of clinical health and medical information resources, hospital librarians assist patients and their caregivers with finding needed health and medical information related to specific clinical conditions. They also understand or have an appreciation for hospital operations and politics and know how to work within a hospital environment.

Corporate librarians share many of the standard librarian characteristics; however, the clinical context and knowledge skill set for working with consumers and patients may be lacking. Of course, academic health sciences librarians are able to function within a consumer library effectively as they are familiar with hospital environments and clinical information.

Several graduate library school programs are offering specialized courses in medical librarianship and/or consumer health librarianship. In addition, the

Medical Library Association offers a specialization in consumer health information. This specialization is offered at two levels depending upon the depth of knowledge desired, requiring twelve to twenty-four hours of approved course work. More details are available at http://www.mlanet.org/education/chc/.

Non-Librarian Staff

Depending upon where the consumer library is located and how it reports organizationally, hiring non-librarian staff varies by institution; check with the personnel department about hiring procedures. Non-librarian staff may include paraprofessionals and student workers. Volunteers are also a frequent source of labor for consumer health libraries, albeit with the caveats mentioned previously. Sources of volunteers include:

- Alumni of the health sciences' schools, if the library is part of an academic health sciences center.
- From the general community.
- Retired healthcare workers.
- High schools.
- Community service programs.

Policy and procedures documents exist to set performance expectations, educate all staff on patient confidentiality issues, set service parameters, meet accreditation standards, and define appropriate levels of health information provision.

Funding Staff

Consumer libraries can be funded by many different mechanisms and sources. Securing solid funding is critical as it determines how many and what type of staff may be appointed. There may be a mixture of funding sources for a consumer library. For example, typically hospital budgets have direct funds allocated for the library. Some academic health sciences libraries fund consumer libraries as part of their health sciences' centers. Supplementing these funding streams are additional resources that may include private donors as well as support from any number of foundations. When seeking supplemental funding from philanthropic individuals or organizations, consider that consumer libraries provide great opportunities to leave a legacy through the ability to name the library or one of its reading rooms after a donor. Such gifts to the consumer health library may also garner community media exposure, promoting the philanthropic individual or organization. Grateful patients and family members and, in academia, alumni, especially if they use its services and resources, often contribute financial support for consumer libraries. In some cases, state funding may support consumer libraries.

With extramural funding sources' emphasis on health literacy, many consumer libraries can obtain federal or state grants, contracts, or subcontracts to achieve key projects or provide outreach services to the general community. This funding can pilot new services or target groups that are not within the library's primary service audience. Consumer libraries can also consider providing services for a fee to recoup some of their staffing costs.

Bright Lights: A mixture of funding sources enabled the financing of a medical librarian for a new consumer health library at the University of Utah. The George S. and Dolores Dore Eccles Foundation funded a medical librarian for two years in return for annual progress reports. The Foundation supported the consumer library so it could reach out to the general community and be of service beyond hospital patients. This seed funding covered the gap for two years until the library obtained release of previously committed personnel funds.

Regardless of the source of funding, consumer health librarians must be great stewards of monies allocated for staffing by accounting for expenditures and revenues. Annual reports, financial reports for sponsoring institutions, and public recognition of donors provide accountability.

Hiring Staff

What kind of knowledge, skills, and attributes a consumer health librarian needs to possess lies in knowing what populations he or she will serve: health professionals, patients, family members, caregivers, the general public, or a specific subset of these populations (e.g., healthcare providers only). For the purposes of this discussion, the necessary knowledge, skills, and attributes outlined in the following are for hiring a consumer health librarian *not* serving healthcare providers.

Knowledge, Skills, and Attributes

A common required qualification for medical librarians is an American Library Association–accredited master's of library sciences degree, and this holds true for consumer health librarians as well. Other subject degrees may be of great benefit, including social work, nursing, health promotion and education, or any other clinical degree or training. Social work is mentioned due to that fact that many of the questions asked by consumers relate to community support services, discharge planning, financial assistance, and other helpful resources. Understanding medical terminology and clinical knowledge is a plus in providing consumer health information. Work experience in consumer health information, public health, or health literacy is also a plus.

The number of years of experience needed varies upon the extent the librarian will be supervising others, responsible for finances and strategic planning, and how independently they operate the consumer health library. A good rule of thumb is the more independence required, the more years of experience needed. If the librarian will be in charge of leading staff, then demonstrated leadership skills are necessary.

Potential consumer health library managers must have proven ability to offer excellent, proactive service to all users, including collaborative partners. The ability to demonstrate excellent oral and written communication aptitudes, organizational problem-solving skills, and project management capabilities is crucial. Knowledge of health information resources and experience with promoting services and resources are other important attributes. Expertise in web content management is a plus, as many consumer health libraries provide selected information to consumers via web portals. Training experience, particularly one-on-one consulting, is needed for providing educational classes and guiding library staff in the development and provision of relevant presentations. In addition, flexibility and adaptability for work in a fast-paced environment as well as excellent interpersonal skills are key characteristics. If supervision is part of the job responsibilities, look for candidates with demonstrated supervisory experience. If fundraising is an expectation, experience with building and maintaining donor relations is desirable. Other important attributes include commitment to both public and community service as well as to diversity in the workplace. Lastly, a sense of humor always comes in handy!

The Hiring Process

Establishing Job Responsibilities and Descriptions

The first step in hiring consumer health library staff is to define the job responsibilities for the positions to be filled. Librarian job responsibilities will depend upon services offered to specified audiences. Defining the librarian's role within the larger organization is also important. For example, will service on institutional committees, task forces or teams (e.g., patient education team) be required? Is the librarian a member of the hospital or health center's leadership team? Depending upon the context, librarians should talk with administrators from the institution in which the library resides as a first step to establishing job responsibilities and descriptions.

Once the key organizational functions for the librarian(s) are outlined, the description typically includes an itemized list of primary and secondary job responsibilities. The types and variety of services as well as the key audiences for such services will assist in determining the desired skill set. Indicate each skill's level of importance in the job description as either "required" or "preferred" qualifications. Salary ranges will be dependent upon existing compensation programs. Exploring salaries of other consumer health librarians ensures competitiveness with the market; therefore, check the *Consumer and Patient Health Information Section* website for current salary information. List the starting salary along with the statement that the final negotiated salary will be dependent on the successful candidate's educational background and professional experience.

Other key components of a job description or announcement include:

- The library and institution description.
- Reporting structure.
- Library staffing.
- Any required statements, such as equal employment opportunity and affirmative action.
- Applicable benefits with reference to obtain more detailed information.
- Description of the city and state to provide the environmental context.
- Method for submitting an application along with a list of required elements such as reference contact information, curriculum vitae, personal statement of interest, or cover letter.

Advertising

Once a job announcement is prepared from the position description, how does one go about advertising for a consumer health librarian? The process is similar to advertising for any other health sciences librarian position; however, there are additional venues available. Using the professional job announcement services of the Medical Library Association (MLA) is a wonderful way to share an opening. MLA has several position announcement options including print advertisements in their newsletter, *MLA News*; its online job line; and via MedLib-L, MLA's listserv. To reach corporate librarians, the Special Library Association is a great place to announce a consumer library

Bright Idea: Table 6.1 provides a job description for a consumer health librarian for the Hope Fox Eccles Health Sciences Library, University of Utah.

TABLE 6.1
Job Description for a Consumer Health Librarian for the
Hope Fox Eccles Health Sciences Library, University of Utah

University of Utah
Spencer S. Eccles Health Sciences Library
Job Description

Job Title: Associate Director, Hope Fox Eccles Health Library
Academic Rank: Associate Librarian

General Responsibilities:
The associate director manages the Hope Fox Eccles Library. This position leads in support of consumer and patient access to a wide range of health and medical information on behalf of varied communities and constituencies both in the hospital and throughout Utah. It is the role of the associate director to create an environment where diverse health information needs are met in a timely and confidential manner.

Specific responsibilities:
1. Plan, manage, and evaluate all aspects of the health library.
2. Serve as a consumer health information advocate to clinical staff, patients, and family members as well as health literacy partners collaborating with the University of Utah.
3. Participate in all aspects of the health library activities including public/partner consumer health training, UtaHealthNet/web content development, community health initiatives, and marketing of library resources and services throughout University Health Care.
4. Supervise, train, and evaluate all health library staff to ensure exceptional patient experiences.
5. Provide information resources and services for library clientele, whether in-person or virtually.
6. Develop community health information public programs.
7. Oversee rotations for students in all health sciences and allied health fields wishing to gain consumer health information experience.
8. Act as liaison between the library and health educators throughout University Health Care.
9. Create and contribute to written reports and documents.
10. Responsible for own professional development and that of staff supervised.
11. Contribute to professional knowledge base by preparing and delivering presentations and publications.
12. Other duties as assigned.

Required Qualifications:
1. Graduate degree from an American Library Association–accredited library science program or relevant master's degree.
2. Work experience with hospital libraries, consumer health, public health, or health literacy.
3. Proven ability to offer excellent, proactive service to all users, clinical staff, and collaborative partners.
4. Excellent interpersonal and communication skills.
5. Ability to work as a team member and independently.
6. Flexibility and adaptability for work in a fast-paced environment.
7. Commitment to service.
8. Commitment to diversity in the workplace or community.
9. Willingness to seek membership in the Academy of Health Information Professionals.

Preferred Qualifications:
1. Professional work experience in academic health sciences, hospital, or public library.
2. Demonstrated ability in project management and information technology including social media.
3. Knowledge of health information resources.
4. Experience with promoting library services and resources.
5. Expertise in web content management and Web 2.0 environment.
6. Experience with evidence-based information retrieval.
7. Demonstrated organizational and problem-solving skills.
8. Commitment to diversity in the workplace or community.
9. Demonstrated supervisory experience.
10. Sense of humor.

Reporting Relationship:
Reports to the Director of the Spencer S. Eccles Health Sciences Library.

position. To reach public librarians, there is the American Librarian Association listing known as American Library Association Joblist and the Public Library Association's career site (http://www.ala.org/pla/tools/careers). Using the *Association of Academic Health Sciences Libraries* listserv is another excellent means of sharing vacant positions. Inform local, state, and regional library associations, too. Of course, word of mouth or personal referral is an important way of recruiting individuals, and, lastly, for hard-to-fill or critical positions, one can always hire a recruiter.

For filling other staff vacancies, check with the organization's human resources personnel about procedures and policies for hiring staff, including students. Also, confirm volunteer recruitment procedures.

Establishing a Search Committee

When hiring professional positions, most institutions require formulation of a search or screening committee. Often, the names of the committee members are included with the job announcement. In putting the committee together, first check with human resources personnel to determine if a particular committee composition is recommended, such as a mixture of genders, multi-departmental representation, various levels of staff (e.g., supervisory and nonsupervisory or clinical and nonclinical), and ethnicity. Appoint a chair to lead the search committee. The chair's role is to establish and conduct committee meetings and ensure fair review of applicants. Committee training, in the form of mitigating bias as well as affirmative action training, is often a first step. If the librarian's role is to serve on organization-wide committees, consider appointing appropriate representatives to the search committee. For instance, if the librarian provides patient education, then the head of patient education would be a valuable search committee member.

The search committee reviews applications for the preferred qualifications and ranks the candidates. A "criteria checklist" helps ensure fairness in that it outlines how the candidates meet the qualifications and specific information about the individuals.

Interviews

If many qualified candidates result, using telephone or video interviews may help to filter the number of individuals to invite for in-person interviews. These interviews are shorter in length and include structured questions posed by the search committee. Include time for interviewees to ask questions about the position as well as the institution.

In-person interviews will reflect institutional practices and differ between hospital and academic centers. In both academia and hospitals, interviews consist of a reasonable number of candidates, typically three to five individuals. These more in-depth interviews include:

- A meeting with the search committee (again using structured questions).
- Time with:
  - Relevant institutional administrators (including budget personnel).
  - Library staff, if this position is part of a larger staff.

- The individual to whom the position will report.
- A topical presentation by the candidate.
- Library and organization tours.

Candidates should gain a thorough understanding of both the position and the institution upon conclusion of the interviews.

Candidates reaching the finalist status may be invited back for a second interview (if funding permits) to provide them an additional opportunity to explore the context within which they will work as well as to familiarize themselves with the local community, housing, schools, and other social constructs.

Bright Idea: Sample questions for use when interviewing consumer health librarians:

1. Describe your experience with offering consumer health information.
2. What techniques do you use to keep up with technologies that enable the delivery of information?
3. What experience have you had with interacting with the public?
4. Describe your experience assisting patients with finding quality information resources.
5. What do you hope to accomplish in this position personally or professionally?

Offering the Position

Issues usually covered when offering a position include salary, benefits, funding for professional development and associated travel, support for relocation costs, and start date. Standard practice is to document the formal offer in a written letter or a formal contract, if required, and if relevant, include the rank and/or status for faculty appointments. Depending upon institutional standards, obtain signatures as required and document a formal acceptance of the position.

Onboarding

Just as important as recruiting the right individual to work in a consumer health library is orienting and onboarding the successful candidate to ensure the individual remains a satisfied and productive employee. Onboarding sets the stage for the new employee's success within the organization and, done well, helps establish early job satisfaction while illustrating to the new hire his or her value to the organization. Onboarding is not a one-time session but considered an ongoing activity, ensuring that a new employee understands the culture of the institution as well as his or her role with carrying out its mission. Human resources personnel will ensure new staff are properly onboarded into the organization and may have an associated onboarding kit or new employee packet to support this early interaction. Once organizational onboarding is completed, departmental onboarding begins. This local onboarding can include a review of the organizational structure and communications, the obtainment of an email account and equipment, an explanation of performance expectations and measures, and an introduction to staff and key administrators.

In addition to these elements, apprise the new hire of regularly scheduled, required meetings as well as this person's appointments to specific institutional and/or library committees. It's always helpful to explain important communication venues highlighting options for their effective information sharing. Address early on any questions regarding benefits to avoid confusion.

Staffing Issues

One-Person Library

As consumer health libraries must be convenient for patients and family members to use, they often have extended weekday and weekend hours. Covering all these hours can be a challenge. In a one-person library, in order to attend meetings or get out into the community to provide services and build relationships, the library is often left unstaffed or closed. Some libraries have the necessary security systems in place to leave the library open but unmanned. They let users know it is "self-serve" during those times.

> **Bright Lights:** Work with other consumer health librarians in close proximity to arrange coverage. Form a pool of librarians willing to fill in for each other to cover vacations, sick days, or extended absences, or consider lining up a "substitute" librarian for scheduled absences (e.g., business meetings, vacation).

Solo consumer health librarians may feel isolated. They may be the only librarian in their organization, and have no other professionals with whom to collaborate and problem-solve. Becoming involved with regional library consortia, organizations, and associations is a way for solo librarians to find mentors, friends, collaborators, conspirators, and support systems.

Understaffed

One of the most pressing problems facing consumer health libraries is being short-staffed given their service demand. In addition to simply not having enough people, some librarians in hospitals have been assigned unrelated job responsibilities, such as to provide audiovisual services and multimedia support. With less professional time to devote to library work, this effectively contributes to the library's understaffing. Consider better communicating to senior leadership the value of the consumer health librarian in meeting the organization's mission. Also consider training a library practicum student or a group of skilled volunteers to support library services as a stop-gap measure.

Virtual Services

Virtual services are those initiated electronically, often in real time, where users employ computers or mobile technology to communicate with library staff without being physically present. Email is the most common form of this service, along with chat, videoconferencing, and instant messaging. All require staff. While virtual services can potentially be available twenty-four/seven, no consumer health library is open around the clock. Conduct a user assessment to determine the optimal hours and days of the week for this type of service, and then determine the best staffing option.

Bright Lights: Collaborative chat services provide increased service hours for a lower cost. The Veterans Health Administration Library Network Office sponsors a virtual reference service staffed by a group of volunteers from the VA Library Network (VALNET). Librarians on Call is available during regular business hours, and all VA librarians have access to it. VALNET serves veteran inpatients and outpatients, their families and caregivers, VA staff and employees, and students and trainees in affiliated teaching programs.

Hospital Administration Relations

Consumer health librarians in hospitals may find that administrators do not fully realize the value of their skills. While administration may "really like them," they will consider downsizing the library's operations or its staff during tight financial times. During hard economic times, administration may question library budgets, eliminate or reduce staff, or not fill positions when retirements occur. Because of this reality, hospital-based consumer health librarians must work proactively to embed themselves in support of their hospital's clinical and nonclinical services. Volunteering or asking to be placed on essential committees or teams, such as patient education, patient safety, risk management, or health literacy, helps librarians establish their expertise in these mission-critical areas and bolster organizational support for their role and contributions. MLA's Vital Pathways project has helpful information on building administrative relationships for hospital-based consumer health librarians at http://www.mlanet.org/resources/vital/.

Cohesive Team Building

Whether a solo consumer health librarian or part of a large consumer health library staff, team building is essential. The solo consumer health librarian may struggle to develop a sense of "team." However, if a solo librarian has students and volunteers assisting him or her, then *that* is the team! Work hard to find a way to hold monthly meetings, staggering the days and time each month to make it easier for everyone to attend. Consider virtual meetings as well to improve attendance. Schedule team training opportunities or social events to bring everyone together and foster a sense of cohesion.

If the library is blessed with a large staff, there may be territorial issues that create friction. Having clearly defined job descriptions can lessen this threat, while simultaneously emphasizing the ways each person contributes to the collective mission and goals of the library and the organization. As noted previously, hold regular meetings, assigning staff responsibility for participation. Empower staff to work together to find creative solutions for library issues. Foster staff development collectively and individually, and participate in social events to grow the team's ease with one another and its strengths.

Alliances

To raise the profile of the library within its community, focus on building as many alliances as possible. Hospital-based consumer health librarians often work closely with hospital information technology departments, informatics departments, patient or clinical educators, patient safety and quality teams, to name a few, within their organizations. While territorialism might be an issue, more often than not, these alliances are a boon for librarians as others quickly realize the many ways librarians provide support for the work they do, including support for their patients.

For other consumer health librarians, forming library partnerships (e.g., a hospital library with the local public library or health organization) helps grow or maximize services, shares professional expertise, and reaches wider audiences. Of note, many larger public library systems have staff dedicated to consumer health information, making these partnerships feasible.

Bright Idea: Consider all departments within the broader organization as potential library allies. One hospital-based library found the admitting department to be a terrific partner. Admitting staff directed people to the library (located at the back of the same long corridor), held packages, and other many "little things" to assist them.

Performance Evaluations

Just the thought of performance evaluations can send a wave of panic over both supervisors and employees. Consumer health librarians in hospitals may report to non-librarian administrators who may not totally understand what they do, and their annual review may be the one opportunity they have for an in-depth discussion about their work. With so much riding on a single meeting, it is understandable that employees would feel anxious. Likewise, some supervisors dread conducting performance evaluations because they are uncomfortable delivering warranted negative feedback. They would rather avoid conflict and tense conversations with their employees.

With careful thought and planning, performance evaluations *can* be an enjoyable and meaningful process for supervisors *and* employees. Employees want to know if their performance is adequate, stellar, or in need of improvement. A great evaluation process benefits employees by helping them:

- Eliminate uncertainty about their performance.
- Clarify their role within the organization, and confirm whether their daily performance links to organizational objectives.
- Better understand their strengths and weaknesses, identify developmental needs, and plan next steps in their professional career.

Supervisors want to ensure their employees perform professionally and in accordance with organizational standards, policies, and procedures; they need to assess staff members' performance, development, and achievement as they relate to the larger organization. A great evaluation process will benefit supervisors by helping them:

- Increase mutuality and communication, which promotes workplace happiness, employee motivation, and employee-supervisor trust.
- Learn new things about their employees, such as any difficulties they are facing or "hidden" talents they could utilize in the workplace.
- Find the best fit for staff members' skill and expertise.

The Evaluation Process

More than likely, the organization will have an evaluation process in place, with set requirements for standards, frequency, timing, and documentation. Having an established process ensures evaluations are clear, consistent, and fair for all. It's important for supervisors to be familiar with the organization's defined approach well in advance of an actual evaluation.

There are a wide variety of evaluation methods used in academic and hospital settings. Most contain three key elements: goal setting, continuous feedback, and a formal annual review. Regardless of the method used, hone in on these elements to increase the likelihood of a meaningful and fruitful evaluation process for all.

Goal Setting

Everyone knows what a goal is, right? Not so fast. Goals are *not* a list of what is done—they are the outcomes one hopes to accomplish. A vague goal like, "Next year, I will work harder," is not sufficient. Goals must be SMART: *s*pecific, *m*easurable, *a*ttainable, *r*elevant, and *t*ime-bound. A SMART goal might be, "Within the next year, I will increase the number of community health education programs the library offers by 15 percent." In performance evaluations, it is essential that goals link individuals to library and organizational priorities. Goals may relate to continuous job responsibilities, one-time projects, or new library services, but they should always tie into the organization's strategic priorities and be challenging yet attainable. In planning new goals, it helps to understand that reaching them requires corresponding investments of time and energy.

As part of the performance review process, the first goal should always be to carry out the responsibilities as listed in the staff member's job description. After all, the main task for an employee is to do what he or she is hired to do. The evaluation process is a good opportunity to review staff members' job descriptions to ensure they are current and that they accurately reflect responsibilities. Lastly, supervisors must approve and staff members must come to agreement on individual and group goals.

Continuous Feedback

Talking only once a year during the annual review will do little to enhance employee performance and will increase the likelihood of a high-stakes discussion. Employees thrive on feedback because it ensures they are performing according to expectations. If mid-year evaluation is not required, try to incorporate several informal "mini" reviews throughout the year. These mini reviews are a boon to supervisors as they enhance knowledge of employees' skills and abilities. Because annual evaluations require recording detailed information about an employee's total performance, having multiple mini meetings eases this burden. Creating a file for each employee is a common way to keep track of accomplishments, note areas for improvement, and document any feedback provided throughout the year.

Annual Review

Employees need to be actively engaged in their annual review process in order for it to be meaningful. This will obviously include talking, but it might also involve self-assessment, problem-solving, compromising, and collaborating. Likewise, supervisors need to be confident in guiding employees in setting viable goals, handling conflict resolution, and providing coaching and counseling. These skills are not innate, so supervisors should ask their organizations for training if necessary.

Some common criteria used to rate performance are job proficiency, attendance, obtainment of goals, teamwork and interpersonal relationships, initiative and creativity, leadership, and communication skills. If responsibilities and objectives were not met, examine why. Were duties too difficult to understand or interpret? Were goals too difficult to accomplish due to lack of required time? Were necessary resources unavailable? Lastly, the annual review will usually include a discussion of professional development plans. In these plans, employees outline their competencies and any developmental activities needed to address those activities, then seek learning opportunities at regional and national workshops and conferences to attain competency. Pursuing Consumer Health Information Specialization and the Academy of Health Information Professionals certification through the MLA are excellent professional development goals. Supervisors need to be prepared to help staff set reasonable professional development goals and assist in identifying viable ways for staff to achieve them.

Two Academic Consumer Health Librarian Considerations: Student Evaluations and Tenure

As stated earlier, there will be a plethora of student workers in any academic consumer health information setting. Though usually not full-time, nor generally as committed to the library profession or the organization, students like feedback about their performance, too. An annual review will boost their engagement and motivation, and offer an opportunity to discuss problems and possibilities. There will likely be a different evaluation process for students—if none exists, consider creating an informal process utilizing the three key elements: goal setting, continuous feedback, and a formal annual review.

Academic consumer health librarians may have retention, promotion, and tenure evaluations as well. Obtaining tenure will require developing a work plan for the upcoming year with goals covering job responsibilities, service, and scholarship. Review the timeframe for retention, promotion, and tenure, and have work plans approved.

Rewards

Organizations wanting to keep employees engaged reward their achievements. Such recognition boosts morale and motivation, and provides an incentive to perform at the highest level. While financial rewards are certainly a major source of satisfaction and motivation, other factors in a reward system can be equally important, including fostering intrinsic rewards, formal recognition, and support for professional development.

Financial

The most common financial incentive system found in academic libraries and business settings is a performance-based reward system. The success of a merit system depends upon consistent and fair performance standards, so performance evaluation data often help determine these rewards. Businesses also use incentive or bonus pay to reward employees who exceed the objectives and expectations of their performance evaluations.

Intrinsic Rewards

Traditional, extrinsic financial rewards such as pay raises and bonuses are declining. Academic and business settings are focusing instead on fostering intrinsic rewards that result when employees find meaning in their work and do it well. These emotional connections to work can be highly energizing and engaging. Without intrinsic rewards, employees may feel they are making no progress and are likely to become cynical and resentful about their work. Fortunately, consumer health librarianship *is* meaningful work!

Formal Recognition

Many libraries' reward systems include service awards, on-the-spot recognition, and peer-to-peer recognition. Verbal praise, plaques, certificates, or small gifts are often given. Recognition is linked to excellent performance, and praise is tailored to the individual and his or her accomplishments.

Professional Development

Providing opportunities to upgrade skills and interact with professional colleagues is highly valued by employees. This is a win-win opportunity for the organization, too, as staff training and development help employees achieve strategic initiatives. It's incumbent upon supervisors to support their employees' efforts to perform to the highest possible standard, as well as prepare and develop them for more advanced responsibilities. Fortunately, library training and educational opportunities abound through the MLA, *Consumer and Patient Health Information Section*, and the National Network of Libraries of Medicine.

Summary

To summarize, recruiting and retaining talented staff for a consumer health library is one of the most important elements leading to its success. Patients and their caregivers offer unique and challenging opportunities in providing subject-specific information services and support. Interactions and communications between library staff and patients need to be confidential, trusted, and results oriented. Ensuring that staff offer this level of engagement and privacy is key to making individuals feel comfortable with seeking information about their personal healthcare. To ensure top-level consumer health information service is delivered, put great emphasis into recruiting and retaining the best and brightest staff. They truly are the consumer health library's most prized asset.

7

Health Reference Service

Nancy Dickenson, Carmen Huddleston, Jean Johnson,
Gillian Kumagai, and Edgar López

R EFERENCE SERVICE BEGINS WHEN a patron presents with an information
need. A librarian then becomes a bridge, connecting the user to the information resources they seek. These tenets of reference service are the same in all
types of libraries, but the provision of consumer health reference stands apart.

There is a responsibility inherent in consumer health librarianship not
found in other reference work, as patrons' very lives may be at stake. Whether
a patron is a patient or family member, the ultimate goal of searching for
information may be to make a critical decision about choosing treatment or
understanding a diagnosis. The interaction may be fraught with emotion, as
patrons may need to share intimate, even frightening details with a librarian. Add in an ever-changing and complex healthcare system, pervasive new
technology, and a demand for evidence-based research and the interaction
becomes even more daunting. Librarians today face unprecedented challenges when providing consumer health information.

The volume and complexity of medical information is growing just as the
healthcare infrastructure is placing increasing demands on patients to participate in their own care decisions. Despite an omnipresent Internet and the
sense of empowerment that it offers to us all, the need for an evidence-based,
consumer health reference service is as important as ever.

The Internet has changed the face of health and healthcare. Internet use by
adults searching for consumer health information is well documented. While
the Internet provides a ready source of information, the consumer's ability to
understand the content and make an intelligent judgment about the validity
of the information is often inadequate. Research indicates that few are skilled

in Internet searching or skeptical and capable of effectively evaluating the information found (Hersh, 2008). The provision of quality, evidence-based information is critical when consumers are making important healthcare decisions. A professional librarian, well versed in consumer health reference work, can play an important role in helping consumers find scientifically based information from a trustworthy source.

Even so, proving the value of a librarian-mediated search is a challenge. In a world where people believe that search engines hold all of the answers, it can be difficult to explain why it is not always the best solution to "Google" for health information. This is why a successful reference experience is important. It can transform even the most skeptical patron into a fan. The following case study illustrates this point:

> Dorothy came into the library having already done her own research online. Her daughter was diagnosed with a brain tumor, and her daughter's doctor recommended the standard protocol, which included a high dose of radiation. Dorothy worried about the side effects of radiation to a three-year-old brain. She had some sites online that led her to believe that there were places in Europe where children were successfully treated with a much lower dose of radiation. Dorothy was intrigued but had no way to determine if this was a legitimate treatment. Her daughter's doctor was skeptical.
>
> Dorothy showed the librarian the sites she had viewed. The librarian searched PubMed to see if any peer reviewed publications supported the reduced treatment regimen. Indeed, there was an individual doctor in Europe who had published research on the subject. Dorothy received copies of those papers from the librarian and found out how to contact the researcher. She talked to her daughter's doctor, who spoke with the doctor in Europe. Not only was Dorothy's daughter treated successfully with the reduced dose of radiation, it ultimately helped many more children as the protocol for treating similar tumors in children was changed.

Evidence-Based Practice

Evidence-based medicine is the practice of systematically locating, appraising, and applying high-quality research in an effort to make sound clinical decisions (White, 2002). Applying criteria for evidence-based information is critical when helping consumers find the information they need to make decisions about their personal healthcare. Evidence-based practice should be an integral part of providing reference service to the public.

Evidence-based practice is based on two fundamental principles. First, patient values and preferences are an essential part of the decision process; second, the better the quality of the research results, the more confident one can be with a decision. The second principle requires consumers to understand that not all evidence is valid and that there are factors such as the size of the study, the exact methodology for conducting the study, and potential conflicts of interest that can affect the accuracy of the results (Schardt, 2011).

Evidence Online

There are a number of resources available to guide patients and consumers in the evaluation of evidence-based information, including the National Cancer Institute (2012), MedlinePlus (National Library of Medicine, 2012), Health on the Net Foundation (2012), the Medical Library Association (2013), the National Center for Complementary and Alternative Medicine (2013), and the Meriam Library of California State University at Chico CRAAP Test (Meriam Library, 2010). The "Bright Lights" box below provides a list of questions these sources suggest be asked when evaluating online health information.

Bright Lights: Evaluating Online Health Information

1. Who manages or sponsors the website?
   - The URL (.gov, .edu, .org, .com) reveals author or source and may point to bias.
2. How current is the information?
   - Look for last update or dates on documents.
   - Look for broken links, indicating the site might not be kept up to date.
3. Does the information complement and not replace the doctor-patient relationship?
4. Is it evidence-based?
   - Information should be presented in a clear manner and verified from a primary information resource, such as professional literature or links to other websites.
   - If an opinion, it should be dated and identified as such and come from a qualified professional or organization whose name and credentials are shared.
5. Who is the intended audience?
   - Consumer or the health professional?
   - If the resource provides information to both consumers and professionals, the website design should make the selection of the appropriate content area clear to the user.
6. Is personal information protected?
   - Personal information should not be shared unless there are clear policies to protect an individual's privacy.
7. Feel skeptical about the site?
   - Check more than one source.

The Reference Interview

It is challenging to conduct a skillful consumer health reference interview. A patron may have difficulty understanding medical terminology, be emotionally frail after a new diagnosis, or be hesitant about communicating a personal issue (Eberle, 2005; Price, Urquhart, and Cooper, 2007; Thomas, 2005).

Users frequently have a difficult time expressing their specific information needs. Dewdney and Michell write: "Librarians have long recognized the tendency of library users to pose their initial questions in incomplete, often unclear, and sometimes apparently covert terms" (Dewdney and Michell, 1997, p. 51).

Anxiety about a condition, embarrassment about discussing personal issues, and lack of understanding of a diagnosis are just a few of the many reasons why users may struggle to express their health-related questions. Through the reference interview, the librarian can help the user clarify and define the specific information he or she is seeking. This, in turn, enables the librarian to provide the most relevant materials in response to the query.

According to the National Network of Libraries of Medicine, some of the special circumstances that a librarian may encounter during a consumer health reference interview include the following:

1. Consumers have incomplete information about their health condition or are unfamiliar with the terminology.
2. Information needed may be of a sensitive nature, such as a sexual or mental health condition.
3. A patron may feel nervous, embarrassed, upset, or emotional, and health concerns may be serious, life-altering, or life-threatening. Often the individual or a loved one is newly diagnosed.
4. Consumers may have unreasonable expectations about the information available. For instance, they may want an easy-to-read resource that clearly explains their medical condition or a straightforward answer to a complex medical question. In reality, this kind of information may be difficult or impossible to find.
5. Consumers may be concerned about confidentiality, anonymity, and security, especially about their personal health information transmitted electronically.
6. Consumers may be confused about the role of the librarian. They might assume that the librarian can advise them on making healthcare decisions.
7. Librarians may be afraid of providing the wrong answer to the individual's health information question, or be concerned about providing negative information to the patron (Ham and Liebermann, 2012).

Regardless of collection focus or community served, the reference interview is of critical importance to all librarians. In all types of reference interviews, the librarian should:

- Demonstrate a welcoming presence.
- Show interest.
- Allow the patron to express him- or herself without interruption.
- Use open-ended and neutral questions to solicit information.
- Verify that the information given is what is needed.
- Close by encouraging the patron to ask future questions (Eberle, 2005; Price, Urquhart, and Cooper, 2007; Thomas, 2005).

Steps of the Consumer Health Reference Interview

In addition to the patron's general contact information, initial information intake should also include age or age range, gender, other existing health conditions, called comorbidities, as well as treatment. Age and gender are important factors when reviewing resources on a condition or treatment. Published research and medical reference materials may categorize the results and treatment options based upon these criteria. Knowledge of other existing conditions and treatment is also important when interviewing a patron. Literature may cover comorbidities, and concurrent treatment that may have an impact on the research request.

Another important determination is: who is the information for? Library patrons may request information on behalf of a relative or friend, as well as for themselves. They may be working on a school report or simply curious. Patrons may provide their own gender and age, but neglect to tell you the information is for someone else.

What level of information do they want? During the interview, try to determine patrons' health literacy level. Showing examples of professional-level versus consumer-level materials is useful when describing the type of resources available. A good health literacy benchmark would be to ask the question, "What type of material would you prefer: written or something visual?"

Knowing the patron's level of understanding can establish a baseline the librarian can use to determine appropriate information for the patron. Therefore, it is always good to ask, "How much do you already know about the condition or treatment, and how did you learn about it?" It is dangerous to assume that a patron is familiar and comfortable with his or her health condition unless he or she demonstrates that understanding. Presenting information on a sensitive subject to an unprepared patron can be distressing for all parties concerned, so ascertaining how much they know already is crucial to avoid this misstep.

Patrons may already have information from a healthcare provider or from the Internet, so clarify this by asking. Doing so can avoid duplication of effort and may also provide insight into what the patron is really seeking. When an individual has already done a lot of Internet searching, find out about the specific websites he or she visited. Whenever possible, offer these individuals additional appropriate websites that may supply the desired information.

To aid successful communication between patron and consumer health librarian, which is crucial to the success of the reference process, a checklist approach can be used. A well-executed reference interview that follows the flow and structure of a checklist can help the librarian delve into the deeper aspects of the individual's information concern and positively influence the outcome of a complicated interaction (Coonin and Levine, 2013). Table 7.1 shows the Research Request Form used as a checklist during reference interviews at Stanford Hospital Health Library (Stanford Hospital Health Library, 2013).

Getting to the Real Question

Patrons may not be fully aware of how to articulate the information they want or need. They may ask a question and during the interview process it becomes evident the information they are really seeking is on a different issue. Often in the medical center setting, the library is the first contact for more information on a diagnosis. Patrons may be confused, upset, and not know how to ask for what it is they are seeking. They may not know what to share because they do not know what is relevant to the interview and subsequent research.

To overcome this, listen carefully to what the patron is saying. Allow the patron to fully state his or her request in his or her own words. Try to avoid influencing what the patron is asking (Reference and User Services Association [RUSA], 2010). Write down exactly what the patron says, using his or her words. A patron may not know how to say or spell medical terminology. It may be a word that is also unfamiliar to you. If so, a medical dictionary can provide the meaning and put the condition into a larger context in order to begin the research process.

After the initial reference interview, repeat the patron's question to verify that correct information has been collected. Doing so allows the patron the opportunity to confirm or perhaps rephrase the original request. Say, for example, "I understand you want to know more about treatment choices for atrial fibrillation, is that correct?" Michele Spatz, in *Answering Consumer Health Questions*, calls this the "talk-back" or parrot technique (Spatz, 2008).

TABLE 7.1
Stanford Health Library Research Request Form

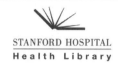

STANFORD HOSPITAL
Health Library

RESEARCH REQUEST FORM

NAME_____DATE_____

ADDRESS_____

_____STATE_____ZIP_____

PHONE NUMBER_____FAX_____

EMAIL _____
(PLEASE READ BACK TO CALLER TO CONFIRM ALL OF THE ABOVE)

INTERVIEWER NAME: _____
********************* *Fold from top to here to protect Patron Privacy* ****************************
Notes from Reference Interview (WRITE ON BACK IF YOU NEED MORE SPACE):
IS THIS INFORMATION FOR : SELF / OTHER_____

PATIENT AGE _____   PATIENT SEX: M / F

Information to be: ☐EMAILED ☐FAXED ☐POST-MAILED ☐NO PREFERENCE

Body Part Affected:

Diagnosis:

Stage of Disease or Prior Treatment:

What is Your Question? _____

_____

_____

KIND OF INFORMATION DESIRED AND LEVEL OF DETAIL
☐ General information—includes definition, diagnosis, care, and treatment
☐ Latest research   ☐ Support groups and/or local agencies
☐ Patron just starting research or   ☐ Patron has some prior knowledge of topic(s)

PACKET COMPLETED BY _____ DATE_____
PLEASE CHECK HERE IF YOU HAVE ALREADY EMAILED OR FAXED THE INFORMATION REQUESTED ☐
Have you answered the question? Yes___ No___(if no, please explain—use back if needed) v.8-6.16.13

While it is important to encourage conversation, librarians should never share their personal experiences or offer advice.

Clarifying questions and reflective listening techniques can show empathy and compassion. Ask open-ended questions to encourage a patron to expand on the information provided. Think about the "Five Ws," an adage commonly used in journalism. Ask "who, what, when, where, and why" when conducting the interview.

One can also take advantage of an opportunity to teach that is unique to in-person reference (Spatz, 2008). For example, before beginning in-depth research for a patron, the librarian can say something like, "So you would like to understand your atrial fibrillation better? Let's take a look at a website called MedlinePlus and find out more." Or, "While I look online for answers to your question, here is a book on heart arrhythmias that you might find interesting."

After the patron reviews the materials, subsequent questions may arise. Let the patron know he or she can return to the library if additional questions arise. Always close a reference interview with an invitation to ask for more.

Reference Challenges

Understanding an individual's real information need does not mean that a satisfying answer will be found. This is part of the challenge of reference work. Perhaps published research on the requested topic does not exist. For example, there are no currently published studies on the effects of using underarm deodorant on the entire body or of life expectancies of ovarian cancer survivors after ten years in remission. Unfortunately, the librarian does not realize information is elusive until after having spent a great deal of time and effort looking for it. In these cases, it's important not to get discouraged and to remember that finding no research is itself significant information. It may not be either the librarian's or the patron's favorite response, but it still is a legitimate answer.

Another challenging reference request comes when a patron asks a librarian to prove a negative. For example, a patron asks for evidence that drinking carbonated water does not cause migraines. This request may require that the librarian spend a lot of time sifting through voluminous literature on migraines, hoping to find the one study that may have looked at carbonated water as a possible trigger. After much research, the librarian may determine that such a study doesn't exist, meaning there is no written statement concluding "carbonated water does not cause migraines." In this situation the librarian can respond by providing the patron with sources that list known migraine triggers, then letting the patron discover carbonated water is not included.

The lack of clear communication between patients and their care providers may pose a difficult scenario in the reference setting, especially when patients leave their provider's office not fully understanding the ramifications of a diagnosis. For instance, a young man might come to the library for information about brain tumors and treatment for his recently diagnosed wife. As he starts going through the reference material, he may become very distressed because no one had told him his wife's "tumor" meant she had "cancer." Unfortunately the library becomes the place where the husband first heard this vital news rather than in the doctor's office where he and his wife could ask specific questions about this frightening diagnosis. In such circumstances, it behooves the librarian to offer comfort care to this individual in the form of a listening ear or encouragement to contact the care provider for a more thorough conversation about the cancer diagnosis.

Challenging reference interactions are illustrated in the following example:

> Pearl was pregnant and diagnosed with breast cancer. She was understandably concerned about the effect of cancer treatment on her unborn child. She came into the library hoping to find research articles that reported successful outcomes in patients like her who opted not to have chemotherapy.
>
> Librarians could not find any published literature that showed successful outcomes for Pearl's type of breast cancer when either a placebo was given or treatment was declined. Although Pearl did not receive the search results she hoped for, she was grateful to receive current articles on management of pregnancy-associated breast cancer.

Types of Reference Interviews

The evolution of communication technology continues to impact consumer health reference work. Classic face-to-face interaction may be optimal for receiving the most complete range of communication cues and informing the reference interview; however, other formats for submitting questions and conducting reference services are becoming more common. Telephone, e-mail, and live chat are important modalities in consumer health librarianship.

Librarians interact with users in various ways but no matter how the information is exchanged, there are shared elements of the reference transaction intersecting all types of communication. Table 7.2 highlights both similarities and differences found in reference interactions, based on mode of communication (Dickenson and Kumagai, 2013).

TABLE 7.2

Health Reference Process by Mode of Communication

	Set the Stage	Gather Facts	Ask and Ask Again	Give Information	Verify	Open Closure
In person	Position the service desk in a prominent place. At the desk, look up, make eye contact, use welcoming body language, and have a friendly expression.	Greet user in a personal and comfortable way (e.g., "Hi, may I help you?"). Restate what you have understood of user's questions. If necessary for a shared understanding, paraphrase.	The initial question may not be the real question. Use open-ended questions to determine patrons' information needs and health literacy.	Turn computer screen towards user and include him or her in the search. Let the user know what you are looking for and why.	Before searching, restate the question in your words to confirm the request.	When you think you have answered the question and have delivered information to patrons, ask them if their questions have been answered. Always invite them to come back and ask more!
Email	Display chat link prominently on all web pages. Let users know when questions can be submitted (or if service is twenty-four/seven).	Give users a personal greeting along with the scripted greeting. Use first names if possible (e.g., "Hi, Pat, that's an interesting question.").	The initial question may not be the real question. Use open-ended questions to determine patrons' information needs and health literacy. Don't be afraid of back and forth communication, despite email's lack of immediacy.	Use the reference request form to explain why the patron's responses will help you provide a more helpful answer. You may need to repeat that message in subsequent emails.	Before searching, restate the question in your written words to confirm the request.	When you think you have answered the question and have sent information to patrons, send an email to ask them if their questions have been answered. Always invite them to email again and ask for more!
Virtual/online	Provide an easy-to-find and well-designed form that is not overcrowded. Questions can be submitted twenty-four/seven.	Send an automatic receipt thanking the user for the question and explaining when a response can be expected.	The initial question may not be the real question. Use open-ended questions to determine patrons' information needs and health literacy. Don't judge patron needs based on chat skills.	Keep patrons engaged in the conversation. Ask if they received the page you sent. Ask if the information is the sort of thing they want.	Before searching, restate the question in your words to confirm the request. Send something that you think will be useful and ask if it's on the right track.	Before ending the virtual interaction, ask if the patron's information need has been satisfied. Invite them to return if they have more questions.

Telephone

Long before the prominence of email and chat, the telephone enabled libraries to serve remote users. Today the phone still affords great opportunities to connect with users who may not be able to come to the library or those who cannot or choose not to access the library through electronic means. Nonetheless, telephone reference has its limitations.

Callers often want the answer to a reference question over the phone, yet responses to some queries do not lend themselves to this format. It is not practical to read complete articles over the phone, and one cannot give incomplete information. Medical words are frequently misunderstood. So while librarians can respond to inquiries about their collection, provide information about local resources, and answer other ready reference type questions, they should not relay medical information beyond a simple definition over the phone. It is acceptable to read a definition from a dictionary, provided the source is always cited. For those callers whose questions cannot be answered by phone, the librarian may suggest the user come into the library. If the person is unable do so, the librarian may offer to mail or email materials after conducting a reference interview.

Virtual Reference

Virtual reference is well integrated into library services and has been since the advent of email reference. The RUSA states, "Virtual reference is reference service initiated electronically, often in real-time, where patrons employ computers or other Internet technology to communicate with reference staff, without being physically present. Communication channels used frequently in virtual reference include chat, videoconferencing, Voice over IP, cobrowsing, e-mail, and instant messaging" (RUSA, 2010). RUSA's "Guidelines for Implementing and Maintaining Virtual Reference Services" offer a helpful framework, and even those experienced in virtual reference may benefit from evaluating their reference services against these guidelines.

Email

Email reference allows users to contact the library without the constraints of geography or time. In order for asynchronous communication to be effective and efficient, one must consider how to best shape these interactions.

While the library's email address is no doubt included in the contact information, it makes sense to have a web form specifically for reference questions. The form serves as the reference interview and consequently it is important to choose questions that will solicit the information needed to begin research, in addition to providing a statement of the library's scope of service. It should be made clear to users that their answers to the web form's questions will help ensure the information they receive back is most relevant to their specific concern. One may consider the following questions for a web form:

- What is your age and gender?
- What is the diagnosis?
- How much do you already know?
- What is your question?
- How do you plan to use the information we send?

No matter how well the form is designed, the librarian will frequently have to engage in a back and forth exchange for question clarification. This exchange often lacks the immediacy of a face-to-face and/or telephone conversation in that email communication can be marked by large time gaps between responses. Some may find it is easier to contact the user by phone to clarify their question.

Bright Lights: The following example is from an email request received by the Stanford Hospital Health Library:

> Can you send me as much research as you can on arthritis? Anything regarding the cause, most successful treatments, etc., would be appreciated.

Where to begin? Because the question is so broad, the librarian must first educate the requestor on the basics of the topic, arthritis, and the library's services before providing more detailed information. Part of the initial response to this request was:

> This email includes a full-text document that describes different types of arthritis. In order to locate appropriate research and studies, we would need to know the specific type of arthritis and which joints are involved. We've also included several research article abstracts. This is a sample of the type of information we can provide.

The hope is that the patron writes back with more details on the diagnosis or what specifically he or she is looking for. Even if the patron doesn't respond, the librarian can find some solace in providing the patron with a more informed beginning for his or her own research.

Chat

Chat offers another option for remote users. These exchanges are convenient for users as their experience is interactive and responses to queries are in real time.

Staffing is a major consideration when undertaking a chat reference service. It is not realistic for the librarian at the reference desk to respond to both chat and face-to-face requests. Due to the real-time nature of chat, the efficacy of the librarian's efforts is dependent on a singular dedication to that specific chat exchange. This efficacy diminishes if the librarian needs to help other individuals at the same time. Though chat may be a viable method of communication, the bottom line is that it is difficult to maintain a chat service unless someone's position is dedicated to respond to virtual requests or the responsibility is shared among staff scheduled for specific shifts to field chat queries.

There are many options when choosing chat reference tools. Free instant messaging tools may meet the needs for basic reference transactions. Libraries that want greater functionality such as co-browsing with the user can purchase proprietary software. Software options are constantly changing. The American Library Association's Technologies Toolbox (http://www.ala.org/rusa/vrc/tech/toolbox) offers a comprehensive list of options for providing virtual reference services including collaborative services, chat tools, reference specific tools, and complimentary tools.

Questions asked during chat sessions cannot always be fully answered during the exchange due to the complexity of the questions or the limits of the library's electronic resources. The licensing and copyright agreements of the collection will dictate what may be sent electronically. In general, items found on the Internet are safe to send. The ability to send journal articles electronically is governed by subscription agreements. As is true with other forms of remote communication, the librarian may need to complete the request by offering to send items by post mail.

Taking Library Reference Service to Patients

Following the principles of embedded librarianship, which is taking reference service out of the physical library and going where the patrons are, consumer health library services in some medical centers are expanding to include patients who may not be able to physically visit the library. Patient mobility is an obstacle to library access, and there are additional factors that make a strong argument for incorporating the moveable library model into reference service delivery. No matter how well we market our libraries, it is likely that many patients do not know they exist. Other nonusers may know about the library but lack awareness of its services, think the library is for staff use only, or feel intimidated about coming in and asking for help. Taking the library to patients eliminates these barriers. With the movement towards patient-centered care, it is imperative health information services travel outside the library to the bedside or clinic setting to serve this population.

Bright Lights: Sharp Memorial Hospital in San Diego, California (Davis, 2011), and Englewood Hospital & Medical Center in Englewood, New Jersey (Lindner and Sabagh, 2004), have both implemented programs in which library staff and volunteers provide reference service at the bedside. A similar program has been started at Stanford Hospital & Clinics that will also include outpatients at the Stanford Cancer Institute (Kumagai, 2013).

Providing a mobile reference service is in many ways the same as any other form of reference. The primary difference is that it is a "cold call." Patrons did not decide to make contact with a library themselves and they are not expecting to see a librarian. That means that it is important to describe the library services available to them, perhaps even show some samples of the types of printed or other information they would receive. It is also crucial, in any kind of patient care setting, to carefully observe privacy regulations, especially to ask permission and question cautiously when others are present in the room.

Mobile reference provides an opportunity for librarians to further develop relationships with clinical staff. First of all, it is important for clinical staff to support the mobile library concept. Obtaining their "buy in" before launching a program is critical. Staff can provide patient lists and suggest patients or family members that they think would appreciate contact from the library.

In serving hospital inpatients, turnaround time is important. Patients may be discharged before the information they requested gets back to them. It is a good idea to respond as quickly as possible and include an invitation to contact the library for more information if desired. Obtaining name and address during the reference interview is a good idea so that the information can be mailed to the patient's home in the event they are discharged prior to receiving library resources.

Confidentiality, Privacy, and Scope of Service

All ethical librarians practice the principle of patron confidentiality, but never is it more important than in the interactions regarding personal medical research. At medical and consumer health libraries, a patron's confidence in librarian discretion is paramount. Health librarians often hear many intimate details of someone's health history.

When consumer health librarians do their job right, they listen carefully and non-judgmentally, asking questions to ascertain the appropriate information as well as to keep the patron focused. In responding to patrons' requests, librarians need to be ever mindful of not giving medical advice or opinion, and must sometimes remind patrons of the nature of their role as information liaison, not medical practitioner. In order to avoid misunderstandings about the library's services, it's important to delineate its service parameters. This may include clearly indicating:

- Who can use the service? Is it open to the public or restricted to patients, family members, and those affiliated with the institution?
- What types of questions will the library answer?
- Are the services free?
- What is the typical response time?
- What is the privacy policy?

Guidelines and Caution Statements

Guidelines and disclaimers can help clarify the library's role and responsibility in providing health information. Guidelines refer to rules of practice for staff; disclaimers, also known as caution statements, outline the library/librarian's role, as well as the limits of their responsibility for patrons. Several examples of both of these are listed in Table 7.3 (Ham and Lieberman 2012; Nebraska Library Commission, 1998; University of Connecticut, 2000). Guidelines can provide the librarian and other library staff with an informed beginning to reference service.

Assessing Health Literacy

An effective reference interaction includes a librarian assessing the patron's health literacy. Health literacy is defined in "Healthy People 2010" (U.S.

TABLE 7.3
Guidelines and Caution Statements

Healthnet-Connecticut Consumer Health Information Network. Guidelines for Providing Medical Information to Consumers.
  http://library.uchc.edu/departm/hnet/guidelines.html

Medical Library Association Consumer and Patient Health Information Section. Disclaimers.
  http://caphis.mlanet.org/chis/disclaimers.html

National Network of Libraries of Medicine. The Consumer Health Reference Interview and Ethical Issues.
  http://nnlm.gov/outreach/consumer/ethics.html

Nebraska Library Commission. Guidelines on Medical Questions.
  http://nlc.nebraska.gov/Ref/STAR/chapter9b.aspx

Department of Health and Human Services, 2010) as "the degree to which individuals have the capacity to obtain, process, and understand basic health information and services needed to make appropriate health decisions." Understanding an individual's health literacy allows librarians to find and provide appropriate materials that will answer patron questions and satisfy their information needs.

It is estimated that nearly half of all Americans are functionally illiterate when it comes to dealing with healthcare issues. Functional literacy is needed to be able to read and understand patient consent forms, medication information, and other written health information. Studies of online health resources have found these materials require average reading levels ranging from tenth grade to college (Adult Basic Education Florida, 2013; National Cancer Institute, 2013; Rudd, 2004; Rudd, Pereira, and Daltroy, 2005).

It can be difficult to assess a patron's health literacy during a reference interview. People with low levels of health literacy may be embarrassed to tell a librarian they do not understand. People with stronger literacy skills generally are comfortable asking for more in-depth or professional information (Kars, Baker, and Wilson, 2008).

There are, however, a few clues that may identify patrons with low literacy issues. These patrons might ask poorly worded or vague questions that demonstrate limited understanding of the situation. They may not even look at the material you gave them, saying they forgot their glasses or they tell you they want to look at the information at home (Osborne, 2005).

Some tips to help a librarian assess for health literacy include the following:

- Explain that medical terms are complicated and many people find the words difficult to understand. Ask if the patron ever needs help filling out forms, reading prescriptions, insurance forms, and/or health information sheets.
- Let them know that a lot of people have trouble reading and remembering health information because it is difficult. Ask if they have ever had this problem.
- Offer different avenues to access health information. Ask about their preferred method of learning something new: watching a video, listening, talking with people, or reading.
- Use plain language and avoid medical jargon and terminology (Cornett, 2009).

Language Issues

The challenges of the health reference interview increase when the issue of language is added. Hispanic and Asian populations are currently the fastest growing ethnic groups in the United States (U.S. Census Bureau, 2011). By 2060, it is projected that one out of every three U.S. residents will be of Hispanic origin (U.S. Census Bureau, 2012).

Spanish language consumer health information is readily available. While there is a growing body of consumer health information in languages other than Spanish and English, it is still somewhat limited. The Cross Cultural Health Program in Washington produced a comprehensive report on access to information that is culturally and linguistically appropriate for all (Cross Cultural Health Care Program, 2007). In addition to their own resources, they cite several organizations as good sources of useful printed and visual material:

- Ethnomed.org: http://ethnomed.org.
- Spiral: http://spiral.tufts.edu.
- 24 Languages Project: http://library.med.utah.edu/24languages.
- NN/LM Consumer Health Information in Many Languages Resources: http://nnlm.gov/outreach/consumer/multi.html.

Communicating with patrons when English is not a patron's preferred language is difficult. Even when there is a bilingual librarian, there can be challenging situations. Patrons may speak in English, even when it is not the language they are most comfortable speaking, simply because they may feel that is expected. It is incumbent upon the librarian to let the patron know they can request library resources and materials in their preferred language.

Of course, the value of any print material is dependent upon the reading level of the patron, independent of language spoken. Even easy-to-read material might be too difficult for patrons who read at a very low level. Audio and video formats, along with photographs or line drawings, can provide a solution when language access or literacy issues present a problem.

Health Librarians Support Clinical Practice

Although the Internet serves as a primary source of health-related information for many patients, most people still consider physicians and caregivers their best source of *reliable* information (Hesse et al., 2005). Health librarians serve both worlds by bringing trusted information resources to patients in the healthcare setting. This allows the caregiver to focus on treating the patient rather than having to locate educational resources for each specific condition in a language and level the patient will comprehend.

"Information prescriptions" are gaining popularity as a way of addressing this need. The healthcare provider fills out a form similar to a drug prescription, but the prescription is for health-related information (Kars, Baker, and

Wilson, 2008). Clinicians who use the information prescription in collaboration with a health library are giving their patients access to trustworthy, evidence-based medical information.

To improve communication between patient and provider, public agencies and private organizations have developed patient guides for talking with healthcare providers. Table 7.4 lists some print, electronic, and video resources to help patients develop questions (Agency for Healthcare Research and Quality, 2012; MedlinePlus, 2013; Joint Commission, 2013). Many of these resources suggest patients ask their physician where they can obtain more information.

TABLE 7.4
Helping Patients Talk to Healthcare Professionals

Agency for Healthcare Research and Quality
http://www.ahrq.gov/patients-consumers/patient-involvement/ask-your-doctor/index.html
  This webpage tells patients how to talk to their professional caregivers. The materials include videos and online and printable lists to help patients prepare questions before their visit, ask during the visit, and then write down any questions that come up after the visit.

The Joint Commission
http://www.jointcommission.org/assets/1/18/speakup_understanding.pdf
  A series of brochures called *Speak Up* encourages patients to ask questions. Patients are told about the right to receive health information in their language and to have a medical interpreter available to explain the caregiver's instructions. There is a link to both the Medical Library Association and MedlinePlus for further information.

MedlinePlus, "Talking with Your Doctor"
http://www.nlm.nih.gov/medlineplus/talkingwithyourdoctor.html
  "Talking with Your Doctor" includes online resources about talking with a healthcare provider. There are links to information in twelve languages, including a video in American Sign Language.

These materials are also beneficial to the consumer health librarian, as they can be used to help patrons formulate and express their information need, thus improving the reference interview. To make these resources more accessible, printed versions of the guides may be distributed throughout inpatient and outpatient settings.

Librarians' Value Is in Building Relationships

When discussing the value of consumer health reference service, librarians are quick to draw attention to resources that take the user beyond Google and the free Internet. While these databases, print books, and eBooks are rich in their offerings, this narrow focus overlooks the most powerful asset: relationships. The importance of what librarians do is not only based upon the pertinence and relevancy of the information they provide but also on their connection with users. The often overlooked value-added is the human element: librarians who listen to the user's needs, define queries, perform searches, and deliver information that will best answer patrons' questions.

In contrast to the algorithmic search formulas employed by Google, Amazon, or Facebook, a good librarian is capable of independent thought. He or she is also committed to nurturing critical thinking in others. Regardless of the technology developed and deployed, librarians provide an often needed human interface to help individuals find their way (Goodyear, 2013). It's incumbent upon librarians to understand how to best foster and maintain relationships with their patrons, so that both clinicians and the public consider them as indispensable partners in the patient experience.

In order to meet their patrons' expectations and foster positive relationships, it behooves librarians to consider the user experience in the design and execution of all reference interactions, whether by telephone, online, or in-person. Regardless of medium, it's important for users to feel welcomed and understood, setting the stage so to speak, so they are comfortable asking sometimes difficult and often highly personal questions. Ending all reference communications with a warm invitation to come back or make contact again if future information needs arise is a positive practice.

Anticipating and being sensitive to patron needs as they navigate their health or medical topic is an important skill as well. For example, while working with a cancer patient, a librarian may learn the individual is adjusting to his or her diagnosis and would benefit from reassuring information resources such as materials on coping, support groups, self-care, and the like. This approach may offer a more comfortable entry point into the vast wealth of consumer health information, especially for someone with a life-threatening diagnosis.

Because clinicians' patients benefit most from the consumer health library's services, librarians are wise to develop relationships with clinicians. Clinicians may not know the breadth and depth of the librarian's capabilities, the extent of the library's resources, or even who it serves. Successful consumer health librarians do not wait for clinical staff to walk in the door to educate them about the library and its services; rather, they seek out opportunities to forge connections. By joining hospital committees, giving presentations at clinical staff meetings, and talking with clinicians one-on-one, librarians share the many ways the library serves and supports patients' ability to learn about their medical diagnosis or condition with evidence-based resources.

Forging clinical relationships is more than just meeting with doctors and nurses and includes social workers, physical therapists, physician assistants, and other clinicians within the larger organization in order to promote the library as a source of trustworthy information.

The value of building strong relationships with patrons is illustrated in the following example:

> Gus initially came to the library looking for a book about heart failure following his wife Elsie's diagnosis. The librarian engaged him in conversation about the library's services, and Gus left with a book along with a number of current articles addressing his specific questions about valve replacement. In a future visit, Gus reported that the articles were instrumental in discussions with his wife's cardiac surgeon. Because Gus and Elsie read the articles, they knew what questions to ask, and his wife was able to successfully have a new minimally invasive procedure with reduced recovery time.
>
> Over the years, Gus has maintained contact with the librarian and has made requests by phone and email for information on other health topics, including his own problems with arthritis. He has repeatedly given feedback that the service he receives from the librarian reduces his anxiety and gives both he and his wife some independence about what the best treatments are when making decisions with their medical team.

Summary

A successful consumer health reference service depends upon many things: solid communication skills, adhering to the components of the health reference interview, and the ability to provide appropriate, evidence-based information in a reading level and language the patron can understand. The advent of new technology continues to change the ways librarians interact with patrons as well as how they find and deliver information.

To thrive in the world of the Internet, with its immediate access to information but often questionable retrieval, librarians must provide consumers and patients with information that is timely, trustworthy, empirical, and highly relevant.

Access to health information empowers consumers, allowing them to participate actively in their healthcare decisions. In today's changing healthcare landscape, it is ever more incumbent upon individuals to understand and be knowledgeable about their own health. Consumer health librarians play an important role, helping patrons navigate the complexity of understanding their medical diagnosis or condition by finding meaningful, evidence-based information that begins with the reference interview.

References

Adult Basic Education Florida. 2013. "Health and Literacy." http://www.abeflorida
.org/healthandliteracy.html. Accessed May 20, 2013.

Agency for Healthcare Research and Quality. 2012. "Questions to Ask Your Doctor."
http://www.aharq.gov/patients-consumers/patient-involvement/ask-your-doctor/
index.html. Accessed May 21, 2013.

Coonin, B, and Levine, C. 2013. "Reference Interviews: Getting Things Right." *The
Reference Librarian*, 54(1):73–77.

Cornett, S. 2009. "Assessing and Addressing Health Literacy." *The Online Journal of Issues in Nursing*, 14(3):Manuscript 2. http://www.nursingworld.org/MainMenuCat
egories/ANAMarketplace/ANAPeriodicals/OJIN/TableofContents/Vol142009/
No3Sept09/Assessing-Health-Literacy-.aspx. Accessed August 12, 2013.

Cross Cultural Health Care Program. 2007. "Culturally and Linguistically Ap-
propriate Health Education Materials: Access, Networks, and Initiatives for the
Future: An Exploration." http://healthequity.wa.gov/Pubs/docs/CCHCP_Rpt.pdf.
Accessed May 20, 2013.

Davis, J. 2011. "For Better Access, Bring the Library Bedside." *Patient Education
Management*, 18(12):138.

Dewdney, P, and Michell, G. 1997. "Asking 'Why' Questions in the Reference Interview: A Theoretical Justification." *The Library Quarterly*, 67(1):50–71.

Dickenson, N, and Kumagai, G. 2013. "Reference Process by Mode of Communication." Stanford Hospital Health Library (2013).

Eberle, ML. 2005. "Librarians' Perceptions of the Reference Interview." *Journal of
Hospital Librarianship*, 5(3):21–41.

Goodyear, S. 2013. "The Future of Librarians in an EBook World." *The Atlantic Cit-
ies.* February 4, 2013. http://www.theatlanticcities.com/technology/2013/02/future
-librarians-e-book-world/4567/. Accessed August 15, 2013.

Ham, K, and Liebermann, J. 2012. "The Consumer Health Reference Interview and
Ethical Issues." http://nnlm.gov/outreach/consumer/ethics.html. Accessed May 18,
2013.

Health on the Net Foundation. 2012. "Looking for Reliable Health Information?"
http://www.hon.ch/HONcode/Patients/visitor_safeUse2.html. Accessed June 5,
2013.

Hersh, W. 2008. *Information Retrieval: A Health and Biomedical Perspective.* New
York: Springer.

Hesse, BW, Nelson, DE, Kreps, GL, et al. 2005. "Trust and Sources of Health Infor-
mation: The Impact of the Internet and Its Implications for Healthcare Providers:
Findings from the First Health Information National Trends Survey." *Archives of
Internal Medicine*, December 165(22):2618–24.

The Joint Commission. 2013. "Understanding Your Doctors and Other Caregivers." http://www.jointcommission.org/assets/1/18/speakup_understanding.pdf.
Accessed May 21, 2013.

Kars, M, Baker, LM, and Wilson, FL. 2008. *The Medical Library Association Guide to
Health Literacy.* New York: Neal-Schuman.

Kumagai, GE. Personal Communication. June 7, 2013.

Lindner, KL, and Sabagh, L. 2004. "In a New Element: Medical Librarians Making Patient Education Rounds." *Journal of the Medical Library Association,* 92(1):94.

Medical Library Association. 2013. "A User's Guide to Finding and Evaluating Health Information on the Web." http://www.mlanet.org/resources/userguide.html. Accessed June 4, 2013.

MedlinePlus, 2013. "Talking to Your Doctor." http://www.nlm.nih.gov/medlineplus/talkingwithyourdoctor.html. Accessed February 24, 2014.

Meriam Library. 2010. California State University, Chico. "Evaluating Information—Applying the CRAAP Test." http://www.csuchico.edu/lins/handouts/eval_websites.pdf. Accessed June 6, 2013.

National Cancer Institute. 2012. "How Can You Be Careful about Cancer Information on Websites, Twitter, YouTube, Blogs, Facebook, and E-mail." National Institutes of Health. http://www.cancer.gov/cancertopics/cancerlibrary/health-info-online. Accessed June 6, 2013.

National Cancer Institute, 2013. "Clear & Simple: Developing Effective Print Materials for Low-Literate Readers." http://www.cancer.gov/cancertopics/cancerlibrary/clear-and-simple. Accessed February 24, 2014.

National Center for Complementary and Alternative Medicine. 2013. "Evaluating Web-Based Health Resources." http://nccam.nih.gov/health/webresources. Accessed June 5, 2013.

National Library of Medicine. 2012. "MedlinePlus Guide to Healthy Web Surfing." National Institutes of Health. MedlinePlus. http://www.nlm.nih.gov/medlineplus/healthywebsurfing.html. Accessed June 5, 2013.

Nebraska Library Commission. 1998. "Guidelines on Medical Questions." http://nlc.nebraska.gov/Ref/STAR/chapter9b.aspx. Accessed June 7, 2013.

Osborne, H. 2005. *Health Literacy from A to Z: Practical Ways to Communicate Your Health Message.* Sudbury, MA: Jones and Bartlett.

Price, T, Urquhart, C, and Cooper, J. 2007. "Using a Prompt Sheet to Improve the Reference Interview in a Health Telephone Helpline Service." *Evidence Based Library and Information Practice,* 2(3):43–58.

Reference and User Services Association. 2010. "Guidelines for Implementing and Maintaining Virtual Reference Services." http://www.ala.org/rusa/sites/ala.org.rusa/files/content/resources/guidelines/virtual-reference-se.pdf. Accessed May 23, 2013.

Rudd, RE. 2004. "Navigating Hospitals." *Literacy Harvest,* Fall:19–24. http://www.hsph.harvard.edu/healthliteracy/files/2012/09/rudd_r.e._2004._navigating_hospitals._literacy_harvest.pdf. Accessed May 20, 2013.

Rudd, RE, Pereira, A, and Daltroy, L. 2005. "Literacy Demands in Health Care Settings: The Patient Perspective." In *Understanding Health Literacy: Implications for Medicine and Public Health,* edited by Joanne G. Schwartzberg, Jonathan B. VanGeest, and Claire C. Wang, pp. 69–84. Chicago: American Medical Association. http://www.hsph.harvard.edu/healthliteracy/files/2013/01/Literacy_demands_in_Healt_care.pdf. Accessed May 20, 2013.

Schardt, C. 2011. "Health Information Literacy Meets Evidence-Based Practice." *Journal of the Medical Library Association,* 99(1):1–2.

Spatz, M. 2008. *Answering Consumer Health Questions: The Medical Library Association Guide for Reference Librarians.* New York: Neal-Schuman.

Stanford Hospital Health Library. 2013. "Research Request Form." Palo Alto, CA.

Thomas, DA. 2005. "The Consumer Health Reference Interview." *Journal of Hospital Librarianship*, 5(2):45–56.

University of Connecticut. 2000. "Guidelines for Providing Medical Information to Consumers." Connecticut Consumer Health Information Network. http://library.uchc.edu/departm/hnet/guidelines.html. Accessed May 18, 2013.

U.S. Census Bureau. 2011. "2010 Census Shows America's Diversity." http://www.census.gov/newsroom/releases/archives/2010_census/cb11-cn125.html. Accessed May 20, 2013.

U.S. Census Bureau. 2012. "U.S. Census Bureau Projections Show a Slower Growing, Older, More Diverse Nation a Half Century from Now." https://www.census.gov/newsroom/releases/archives/population/cb12-243.html. Accessed May 20, 2013.

U.S. Department of Health and Human Services. 2010. "Healthy People 2010: Understanding and Improving Health." http://www.healthypeople.gov/2010/redirect.aspx?url=/2010/. Accessed August 19, 2013.

White, PJ. 2002. "Evidence-Based Medicine for Consumers: A Role for the Cochrane Collaboration." *Journal of the Medical Library Association*, 90(2):218–22.

8

Ethical Issues in Providing Consumer and Patient Health Information

Barbara Bibel with Michele Spatz

COMMITMENT TO INTELLECTUAL FREEDOM and freedom of access to information are core values for librarians. This is especially true when providing health information for consumers and patients. There are special situations that may pose dilemmas for librarians working with patrons needing consumer health information. Those working in libraries affiliated with academic institutions, hospitals, and healthcare systems will sometimes encounter problems that are different than those encountered by librarians working in public libraries. Each has a different mission and a different clientele. There are, however, also common goals and values.

Regardless of library setting, patrons seeking health and medical information may be upset because they or someone close to them has received a diagnosis of a serious condition. They may have incomplete information about it or may not understand the information given to them because they are unfamiliar with medical terminology. Whatever the circumstance, these individuals deserve relevant information at a reading level and in a style that they can understand.

There are a number of things that librarians can do to assure an ethical transaction. Providing a safe, welcoming environment and greeting the person warmly typically helps everyone relax and may improve communication. Where health and medical information is concerned, understanding exactly what the individual needs is crucial and thus the librarian must sometimes ask sensitive questions. It is important to assure privacy and confidentiality when having these important and highly personal conversations.

Some patrons expect things that librarians cannot ethically deliver, such as medical advice. When providing health and medical information, it's important to remember librarians are not licensed to practice medicine and should not do so, even when patrons persist. The caveat here is offer information, not counsel (Charney, 1978). Any time a librarian is interacting with someone seeking medical or health information, the librarian should not offer recommendations nor discuss personal experiences relating to diagnoses, tests and procedures, treatments, outcomes, medical professionals, or institutions.

When sharing information, always cite its source, to confirm its validity. This also helps the patron who wants more detail to know where to look. When sharing information, if applicable, explain that there may be several treatment options for a particular diagnosis or condition, and always encourage the individual to take the information to his or her healthcare practitioner to discuss it. Sometimes patrons will push back against this suggestion, claiming their doctor is too busy to answer questions. This is often a golden opportunity for the librarian to share patient self-advocacy resources—items such as "How to Communicate with Your Doctor" (http://www.nih.gov/clearcommunication/talktoyourdoctor.htm) as well as resources outlining patients' right to a second opinion (http://www.patient advocate.org/index.php?p=691).

As mentioned previously, guaranteeing privacy and confidentiality is a must and a foundational principle of librarianship. Along those lines, if the patron is someone that the librarian knows in another context, the librarian may not inquire about the issue outside of the professional environment. The librarian may not divulge information about *any* patron inquiries. This is stated in the American Library Association Code of Ethics: "We protect each library user's right to privacy and confidentiality with respect to information sought or received and resources consulted, borrowed, acquired or transmitted" (American Library Association, 2008). The Medical Library Association's Code of Ethics for Health Sciences Librarianship also states, "The health sciences librarian respects the privacy of clients and protects the confidentiality of the client relationship" (Medical Library Association, 2010).

There are privacy and confidentiality laws that affect the practice of consumer health librarianship. For example, librarians working in healthcare institutions must adhere to the Health Insurance Portability and Accountability Act of 1996, which protects the privacy of individually identifiable health information (U.S. Department of Health and Human Services, 1996).

The Patriot Act of 2001, which was extended in 2011, impacts all librarians and allows roving wiretaps, searches of business (including library) records, and surveillance of those suspected of terrorist activities. Authorities need a warrant, but no probable cause to obtain one is required. If served with a search warrant, librarians may not disclose its existence or whether any information was provided. Borrower records, Internet logs, and library card registration information may be requested. Librarians should think about the kind of personal information collected on library users as well as how long they retain this information in light of the Patriot Act legislation (American Library Association, 2013).

In all reference work, maintaining an impartial, non-judgmental attitude is essential and this is true in consumer health librarianship, too. Some individuals' questions involve controversial topics. In certain healthcare organizations, there may be institutional policies that forbid the librarian from providing specific types of information (e.g., abortion or birth control information in a Catholic teaching hospital). If possible, referral to an agency that can provide the information is helpful. Sometimes, librarians may have personal religious beliefs that inhibit them from wanting to assist a patron with a request that goes against the librarians' beliefs. Regardless of personal conviction, the librarian is professionally obligated to offer the information or, if there is an option, ask a colleague who is comfortable providing it to assist the patron.

Another dilemma is the patron asking for information about something that may be illegal, such as growing medical marijuana or physician-assisted suicide. Because it is not illegal to learn about these things, the librarian should assist the individual in locating relevant resources. Other topics such as diets and alternative or complementary therapies may also be controversial, and problems exist when one is not able to find impartial, evidence-based resources on these subjects. In these cases, provide information from the best available resources such as professional organizations and agencies, for example, MedlinePlus (http://www.medlineplus.gov), or the National Center for Complementary and Alternative Medicine (http://nccam.nih.gov/).

Providing information about a disease or condition with a poor prognosis can be emotionally draining, especially if the patron is unaware of the situation. When sharing knowledge-based resources with such a patron, the librarian should be supportive but neutral. Encourage patients to discuss their diagnoses with their physician and family. Providing referrals to support groups may be helpful, too. In dealing with distraught patients, those working in libraries in healthcare facilities may have access to social workers and/ or pastoral care. These are helpful, but only if the patron wishes a referral.

One final ethical quandary concerns family members or healthcare providers who may not want a patient to learn about a diagnosis or condition. Yet the librarian's first responsibility is to the patient, whose information requests, privacy, and confidentiality always take precedence, even when the librarian is challenged by family members or other caregivers. If the patron is a child or is mentally impaired, the material should be at the appropriate level of comprehension. Information is an important part of healthcare, and librarians are legally required to provide it when requested (Charney, 1978). Maintaining a current collection, using disclaimers, communicating well, and honoring the accepted standards of library practice are the surest guides for navigating ethically difficult situations.

Summary

While librarians are sometimes met with ethical challenges in providing consumer health information, it does not diminish the valuable assistance and support they deliver to individuals who request their help. The following ethical guidelines support professional practice:

- Be welcoming and supportive, but avoid personal involvement.
- Provide the most appropriate, complete information. Make sure that the language, reading level, and format are suited to the individual.
- Do not diagnose, recommend, or interpret material.
- Maintain privacy and confidentiality.
- Do not offer personal opinions.

TABLE 8.1
Code of Ethics of the American Library Association

As members of the American Library Association, we recognize the importance of codifying and making known to the profession and to the general public the ethical principles that guide the work of librarians, other professionals providing information services, library trustees, and library staffs.

Ethical dilemmas occur when values are in conflict. The American Library Association Code of Ethics states the values to which we are committed, and embodies the ethical responsibilities of the profession in this changing information environment.

We significantly influence or control the selection, organization, preservation, and dissemination of information. In a political system grounded in an informed citizenry, we are members of a profession explicitly committed to intellectual freedom and the freedom of access to information. We have a special obligation to ensure the free flow of information and ideas to present and future generations.

The principles of this Code are expressed in broad statements to guide ethical decision-making. These statements provide a framework; they cannot and do not dictate conduct to cover particular situations.

I. We provide the highest level of service to all library users through appropriate and usefully organized resources; equitable service policies; equitable access; and accurate, unbiased, and courteous responses to all requests.

II. We uphold the principles of intellectual freedom and resist all efforts to censor library resources.

III. We protect each library user's right to privacy and confidentiality with respect to information sought or received and resources consulted, borrowed, acquired, or transmitted.

IV. We respect intellectual property rights and advocate balance between the interests of information users and rights holders.

V. We treat co-workers and other colleagues with respect, fairness, and good faith, and advocate conditions of employment that safeguard the rights and welfare of all employees of our institutions.

VI. We do not advance private interests at the expense of library users, colleagues, or our employing institutions.

VII. We distinguish between our personal convictions and professional duties and do not allow our personal beliefs to interfere with fair representation of the aims of our institutions or the provision of access to their information resources.

VIII. We strive for excellence in the profession by maintaining and enhancing our own knowledge and skills, by encouraging the professional development of co-workers, and by fostering the aspirations of potential members of the profession.

Adopted at the 1939 Midwinter Meeting by the ALA Council; amended June 30, 1981; June 28, 1995; and January 22, 2008. The previous version of this file has long held the incorrect amendment date of June 28, 1997; the Office for Intellectual Freedom regrets and apologizes for the error.

TABLE 8.2
Code of Ethics for Health Sciences Librarianship

Goals and Principles for Ethical Conduct
The health sciences librarian believes that knowledge is the sine qua non of informed decisions in healthcare, education, and research, and the health sciences librarian serves society, clients, and the institution by working to ensure that informed decisions can be made. The principles of this code are expressed in broad statements to guide ethical decision-making. These statements provide a framework; they cannot and do not dictate conduct to cover particular situations.

Society
- The health sciences librarian promotes access to health information for all and creates and maintains conditions of freedom of inquiry, thought, and expression that facilitate informed healthcare decisions.

Clients
- The health sciences librarian works without prejudice to meet the client's information needs.
- The health sciences librarian respects the privacy of clients and protects the confidentiality of the client relationship.
- The health sciences librarian ensures that the best available information is provided to the client.

Institution
- The health sciences librarian provides leadership and expertise in the design, development, and ethical management of knowledge-based information systems that meet the information needs and obligations of the institution.

Profession
- The health sciences librarian advances and upholds the philosophy and ideals of the profession.
- The health sciences librarian advocates and advances the knowledge and standards of the profession.
- The health sciences librarian conducts all professional relationships with courtesy and respect.
- The health sciences librarian maintains high standards of professional integrity.

Self
- The health sciences librarian assumes personal responsibility for developing and maintaining professional excellence.
- The health sciences librarian shall be alert to and adhere to his or her institution's code of ethics and its conflict of interest, disclosure, and gift policies.

TABLE 8.3
Library Bill of Rights

The American Library Association affirms that all libraries are forums for information and ideas, and that the following basic policies should guide their services.

I. Books and other library resources should be provided for the interest, information, and enlightenment of all people of the community the library serves. Materials should not be excluded because of the origin, background, or views of those contributing to their creation.

II. Libraries should provide materials and information presenting all points of view on current and historical issues. Materials should not be proscribed or removed because of partisan or doctrinal disapproval.

III. Libraries should challenge censorship in the fulfillment of their responsibility to provide information and enlightenment.

IV. Libraries should cooperate with all persons and groups concerned with resisting abridgment of free expression and free access to ideas.

V. A person's right to use a library should not be denied or abridged because of origin, age, background, or views.

VI. Libraries that make exhibit spaces and meeting rooms available to the public they serve should make such facilities available on an equitable basis, regardless of the beliefs or affiliations of individuals or groups requesting their use.

Adopted June 19, 1939, by the ALA Council; amended October 14, 1944; June 18, 1948; February 2, 1961; June 27, 1967; January 23, 1980; inclusion of "age" reaffirmed January 23, 1996.
A history of the Library Bill of Rights is found in the latest edition of the Intellectual Freedom Manual (http://www.ala.org/advocacy/intfreedom/iftoolkits/ifmanual/intellectual).

References

American Library Association. 2008. "Code of Ethics." Adopted January 22, 2008. http://www.ifmanual.org/codeethics. Accessed August 10, 2013.

American Library Association. 2013. "The USA Patriot Act." http://www.ala.org/advocacy/advleg/federallegislation/usapatriotact. Accessed August 11, 2013.

Charney, N. 1978. "Ethical and Legal Questions in Providing Health Information." *California Librarian*, 39(1):25–33.

Medical Library Association. 2010. "Code of Ethics for Health Sciences Librarianship." http://www.mlanet.org/about/ethics.html. Accessed August 11, 2013.

Mulac, CM. 2012. *Fundamentals of Reference.* Chicago: American Library Association.

National Network of Libraries of Medicine. 2012. "The Consumer Health Reference Interview and Ethical Issues." Updated by Kelli Ham, July 12, 2012. http://nnlm.gov/outreach/consumer/ethics.html. Accessed August 11, 2013.

Spatz, M. 2008. *Answering Consumer Health Questions: The Medical Library Association Guide for Reference Librarians.* New York: Neal-Schuman.

U.S. Department of Health and Human Services. 1996. "Health Information Privacy." http://www.hhs.gov/ocr/privacy. Accessed February 28, 2014.

9

Social Media for Health Consumers and Patients

Michelle A. Kraft

SOCIAL MEDIA ARE PERVASIVE IN today's culture, used in advertising, journalism, politics, athletics—even disaster planning. Twitter, Pinterest, Facebook, and YouTube have spread beyond the boundaries of websites; the badges of these social media sites can be found on television, magazines, and billboards. During the 2012 Olympics, Twitter and NBCUniversal teamed up, making Twitter an official narrator for live Olympic events. NBC promoted the website during its Olympic programming (Ovide, 2012). Twitter use during the Olympics was so prevalent that it is believed to have interfered with real-time reporting of the cycling events. The large amount of traffic from Twitter jammed the transmission of athlete times and their positions to BBC commentators, leaving commentators to estimate times using a personal watch (Jones, 2012).

Much has been discussed about social media's impact on the uprisings in the Middle East and North Africa; some believe it was the driving force behind the unrest, while others downplayed its impact. While revolutions have occurred throughout history, social media made their communications, shared photos, and personal stories more immediate and widespread than ever. In Tunisia, Facebook posts were the communications medium while in Egypt, Twitter was influential (Beaumont, 2011).

Many individuals report social media, rather than traditional news media, as their most reliable source of information. This was seen in Mexico during its drug wars and also during natural disasters here at home, such as Hurricane Sandy. Damien Cave wrote, "Social media has become a necessity in Mexico, with a mission far different from what has emerged in the Arab revolutions, or in China. In those countries, social networks have been used to route around identifiable sources of repression and to unify groups dispersed over large areas. In Mexico, Twitter, Facebook and other tools are instead deployed for local survival" (Cave, 2011). People use social media to warn others of gunmen, shootouts, drug cartel checkpoints, and other dangerous situations. Cave wrote that news of gunmen holding up rush-hour traffic to dump thirty-five bodies outside of Veracruz, Mexico, was on Twitter before police or reporters were there.

Natural disasters present a different impetus for social media sharing than Mexico's drug wars, but are also about surviving and dealing with the aftermath. During Hurricane Sandy, people used Twitter and Facebook to report on and stay informed about the storm's destruction. The mayor of New York, Michael Bloomberg, @MikeBloomberg, and New Jersey Governor Chris Christie, @GovChristie, tweeted messages about the storm, evacuation routes, and other safety information. According to Sara Estes Cohen, "Hurricane Sandy marked a shift in the use of social media in disasters. More than ever before, government agencies turned to mobile and online technologies. Before, during and after Sandy made landfall, government agencies throughout the Northeast used social media to communicate with the public and emergency response partners, share information, maintain awareness of community actions and needs, and more" (Cohen, 2013). Not only did city and state governments monitor information and answer questions coming from Twitter, Facebook, and Tumblr, but the federal government used social media heavily during the storm. Just prior to Sandy making landfall, a Federal Emergency Management Agency team was watching nearly twenty million Twitter messages about Sandy to monitor the dangerous situation and send out safety information. When Sandy reached land, the Federal Emergency Management Agency reached more than three hundred thousand Facebook followers and six million Twitter users with one message; the word Federal Emergency Management Agency had 5,800 mentions on Twitter per hour, and the agency had more than five hundred thousand visitors to its website Ready.gov (Cohen, 2013). Since then, the U.S. Department of Homeland Security's Science and Technology Directorate established a Virtual Social Media Working Group to provide guidance and best practices on social media use before, during, and after emergencies (Homeland Security, 2013).

Given all of this, it is not surprising people within healthcare have adopted these tools to connect with consumers, patients, and peers. On February 21, 2012, at 5:30 in the morning, Memorial Hermann Health System in Houston, Texas, made history by live tweeting a double bypass surgery. As one doctor performed the surgery, another doctor updated Twitter followers on the procedure and answered questions.

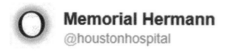 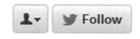

Memorial Hermann
@houstonhospital

Welcome! First LIVE #Twittercast of an open #heartsurgery for the US by Memorial Hermann #hospital in #houstontx #MHopenheart

↰ Reply   ⟲ Retweet   ★ Favorite   ••• More

FIGURE 9.1
The First Live Tweet of Open Heart Surgery from Memorial Hermann Health System

The surgeon wore a camera during surgery and the doctor on Twitter took additional photos, all of which were tweeted, uploaded on YouTube, and added to Storify on the hospital's channels (Laird, 2012). Memorial Hermann Health System continued its foray into social media surgery by subsequently live tweeting and videoing a brain surgery and a c-section delivery. This chapter will discuss the usage of social media to provide outreach to patients and consumers along with areas for its opportunities and growth.

History of Social Media

Starting from the ten day "express mail" services of the Pony Express to the near instant communications of the telegraph's dots and dashes, proceeding to the telephone, fax, and now the Internet, people have always sought to connect to others and share information with greater speed.

In order to fully understand how social media can be used for patient and consumer outreach, it is necessary to define the term "social media" and provide a brief background on its evolution. Thielst defines social media as "electronic tools that enhance communication, support collaboration, and enable users across the globe to generate and share content" (Thielst, 2010, p. 1). These tools are different from traditional electronic communication such as email. Email is usually directed to a specific person or group of people and can only be seen by the people it is sent to. While an email can be distributed beyond the initial recipients, broad distribution is both difficult and limited. Social media tools such as Twitter, Facebook, Pinterest, and Storify are all structured to promote mass collaboration and large-scale communication.

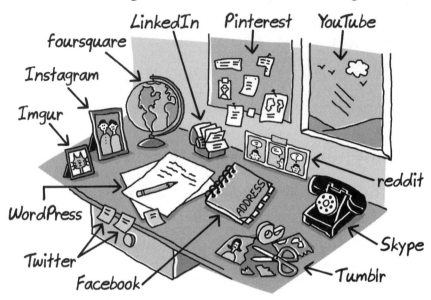

FIGURE 9.2
Vintage Social Networking Cartoon by John Atkinson (http://wronghands1.wordpress
.com ©John Atkinson, Wrong Hands)

Even though there are many social networking tools commonly categorized as social media, these tools are used for various purposes and provide very different ways of interactive communication. Hamm defines five different categories into which social media tools can be grouped: collaborative projects, blogs or microblogs, content communities, social networking sites, and virtual gaming or social worlds (Hamm et al., 2013).

Collaborative Projects

Collaborative projects are tools such as wikis and Google Drive, where content is posted online by individuals but can be modified by others. It is a cooperative endeavor where many people can add, modify, edit, and delete information easily. Wikipedia is probably the most well-known example. Despite controversy over the open editorial nature of the wiki, Wikipedia has grown rapidly since it was created in 2001. As of February 2012, it had 470 million unique visitors monthly, more than eighty-five thousand active editors, and more than twenty-one million articles (Zachte, 2012). Although Wikipedia exemplifies the potentially large extent of wikis, other groups have used wikis to collect and share knowledge among intentionally smaller groups. Diplopedia is the online encyclopedia of the Office of eDiplomacy, Bureau of Information Resources Management of the U.S. Government. It is a tool for State Department personnel needing quick access to helpful and timely information on foreign affairs issues. It grew from ten articles in 2006 to over ten thousand articles in 2010 (Bronk and Smith, 2010, p. 6).

While Google Drive is not as widely accessible as a traditional wiki, it still allows a group of people the ability to share, create, add, edit, and delete documents, spreadsheets, presentations, etc. Google Drive allows groups to collaborate on projects simultaneously and across large distances. The "owner" of the document determines whether the document is available and/or can be edited publicly. The owner can also make the document private, available or edited by certain people or groups.

> **Bright Idea:** Johns Hopkins University School of Medicine used Google Drive as the online resource to house the question and answer sets for the exams in its Genes to Society curriculum. Essentially, they used Google Drive to provide a crowd-sourced study resource for medical students. "In contrast to previous models of distributing course notes, in which a single top performer distributed his or her notes to the entire class, our model relies on a diverse group of students with different strengths and weaknesses collectively creating a public resource" (Bow et al., 2013). Google Drive was chosen because it was familiar to students, user friendly, and allowed multiple people to edit and view documents. The documents were publicly accessible and modifiable, and were shared to the entire class of 2014. "Thus, following the crowd-sourcing model, any student could add material, correct answers, and build custom question sets to aid his or her classmates in understanding the topics. We noticed that some students would write questions and answers in real time during a lecture; other students in the lecture hall would then edit them instantaneously" (Bow et al., 2013).

Blogs or Microblogs

Blogs or microblogs are websites that are typically in a diary type format; entries are arranged by date. Wordpress is a popular blogging platform. Twitter and Yammer are popular microblogs. Microblogs limit authors' posts to 140 characters or fewer. Tumblr can be considered either a blogging platform or a microblog depending on one's perspective. Tumblr does not limit authors' posts to 140 characters, but posts are often much shorter than traditional blog posts. Commonly, one person provides the content for a blog, but there are blogs where a group of people are responsible for writing posts.

Bright Lights: The Medical Library Association's Conference Blog is a good example of a blog with multiple writers submitting posts.

While blogs and microblogs are written by one or a few people, they are considered social media tools because readers have the ability to communicate with the author and other readers. In traditional blogs, readers are able to communicate with the author and other readers by writing and submitting comments to the blog post. Large discussions can go on between author and readers on some posts. For example, the post "I Graduated from a Top Library School. Yeah, So What?" by Joe Hardenbrook on the blog *Mr. Library Dude*, discussing the definition of a "professional librarian" and the difficult library job market, was originally posted July 21, 2011, and has more than seventy comments or responses (Hardenbrook, 2011).

Many of the responses were made within the first month of the original post. However, the discussion continued even one to two years after the original post, with the most recent comment from July 4, 2013.

With a 140 character limit, from a discussion standpoint microblogs are more akin to texting or chatting. Because the message is short, they tend to be a brief post either alone or with a link to news items, thoughts, or perhaps a quick question. While it might seem difficult to hold a discussion with multiple people or share thoughts in only 140 characters, it is quite popular and people "tweet" quite frequently. Twitter has more than a half-billion user accounts and is the second largest social networking site (Lunden, 2012). Twitter definitely can connect people together online, and it may be used effectively in education.

Bright Lights: Several medical librarians use Twitter weekly to learn about various topics of interest. Discussions are held every Thursday at 9 p.m. EST under the hashtag #medlibs. Medical librarians have discussed disaster planning, altmetrics ("alternative metrics," which track the impact of a research article through social media references), and translational science. Transcripts of these discussions can be found at http://medlibschat.blogspot.com/ (Social Media, 2013).

Content Communities

Content communities are websites or tools that allow users to share media content such as videos, photos, and presentations. YouTube, Flickr, Instagram, and SlideShare are all types of content communities. YouTube allows users to share online videos, and registered users may upload an unlimited number of them. YouTube also has different rules for posting videos based upon the type of user account. Regardless of user account type, most posted videos are typically no longer than fifteen minutes. Flickr and Instagram are photo and video sharing services that allow users to post pictures and videos online for others to see. While both are available on the web and mobile platforms, Flickr is more focused on sharing via the web and hosting a photo archive, while Instagram is focused on mobile sharing through real-time feeds. "Figure 1" is similar to Instagram except it is specifically dedicated to medical professionals.

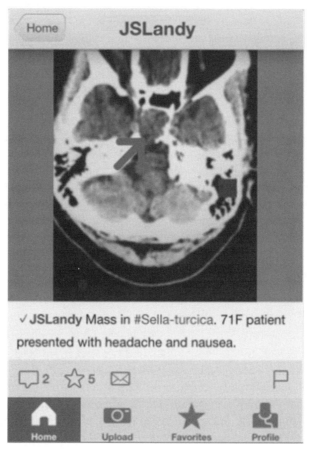

FIGURE 9.3
Screen Shot from Figure 1 App Showing a Mass in the Sella Turcica (©Figure 1, Inc.)

It is a crowd-sourced medical image library for healthcare professionals to share interesting photos with other colleagues. Photos cannot contain personally identifying or patient information. The app includes a consent form and has software that detects faces and automatically blacks them out (Blackwell, 2013). Slideshare is a website dedicated to sharing PowerPoint, PDF, Keynote, or OpenOffice presentations. People may rate, comment, and share already uploaded presentation content.

Social Networking Sites

Social networking sites allow users to create personal information pages or profiles that, depending upon privacy settings, can be accessed by everyone or only by certain groups such as family, friends, or work groups. Facebook, LinkedIn, and Google+ are social networking sites. Facebook is by far the most popular social networking site with 1.06 billion monthly active users and over 1.13 trillion "likes," 219 billion uploaded photos, and 604 million mobile users (Tam, 2013). Facebook tends to have more personal information and people tend to lock down profiles to a select group of friends or family. Posts and pictures are likely to be very personal in nature; Facebook also has online gaming apps and advertising. LinkedIn is geared more as a social media outlet for businesses and professionals. Users create a personal online Rolodex of professional contacts and business associates. There are no gaming apps for LinkedIn, and discussions don't occur on an individual's profile but rather in LinkedIn's groups or communities. Google+ is somewhat similar to Facebook. Users create circles of people they want to follow and with whom they want to share information. Google+ has the ability to allow users to share documents, photos, presentations, etc., through the use of Google Drive and other Google applications. Google+ also allows users to conduct real-time video chats, called Hangouts.

Virtual Gaming or Social Worlds

Virtual gaming or social worlds are sites that replicate alternative worlds. Second Life, created by San Francisco–based Linden Labs in 2003, is an online three-dimensional virtual reality world where users create their own online personalities, called avatars, and interact with others within the online world. Users can visit virtual places, socialize with other users online, and build and create their own objects and places with the Second Life program. The content in Second Life is all user-generated (Gray, 2013). Health Info Island was created through a forty thousand dollar grant from the U.S. National Library of Medicine/Greater Midwest Region of the National Network of Libraries of Medicine to provide consumer health information services in Second Life (U.S. National Library of Medicine/Greater Midwest Region, 2006). Health Info Island was dedicated to providing health information, training programs, and outreach to virtual medical communities, consumer health resources, and one-on-one support to Second Life users (Boulos, Hetherington, and Wheeler, 2007). The Mayo Clinic continues to offer online continuing education courses through Second Life, and the American Cancer Society has used the game to raise more than $1.5 million since 2005 (American Cancer Society, 2012; Kennel, Collazo-Clavell, and Richards, 2013).

The various social media tools illustrate the many different ways people connect to each other as well as to groups to share information and resources. It offers the ability to take consumer health and patient education outreach from a one-on-one interaction to a large-scale, one-to-many opportunity.

Combining Outreach with Social Media

Social media provides librarians and information professionals with a variety of opportunities for reaching consumers and patients. The number of people using social media for health information seems to vary. Thielst reports that 34 percent of health searchers use social media resources to "delve into health and wellness topics" (Thielst, 2010, p. 9). Hamm describes that 72 percent of adults seek medical information online, but only 26 percent were using social media to do so (Hamm et al., 2013). While Thielst and Hamm may have different numbers for the percentage of consumers using social media for health information, they both believe the trend is growing and the percentages of people using social media for health information will increase. Buie attributes the increased usage of social media in healthcare to "the newest consumers of healthcare," Generation X and Generation Y (Buie and Smith Jones, 2011). Not only have these generations grown up with technology, they are the biggest consumers of social media. Pew Research Center reports 83 percent of people aged eighteen to twenty-nine and 77 percent of people aged thirty to forty-nine use social media networking sites (Duggan and Brenner, 2013).

Despite the large number of people seeking health information online and the growing number of people using social media to do so, the effects of social media on consumer or patient health information have not been well documented. Measuring the effects of social media on patient education is difficult at best. Social media supports a transient anonymous style of communication that makes it difficult to measure. Hamm determined the majority of studies on the use of social media in patient and consumer health were descriptive and used content analysis to outline how social media were used. However, he did discover some randomized controlled trials discussing a specific social media tool's impact upon a particular health condition. The majority of these randomized controlled trials related to lifestyle and weight loss, but others pertained to conditions such as tobacco and substance abuse, mental health, diabetes, irritable bowel syndrome, multiple sclerosis, hearing loss, and cancer. In the randomized controlled trials, the social media tool used was just one component in a very complicated intervention, which made determining the tool's specific effect difficult to determine (Hamm et al., 2013). Despite very few studies quantifying the effect of social media on patient education, Hamm et al. states, "Overall, 186/284 (65.5 percent) studies concluded that there was evidence for the utility of social media, while only 15/284 (5.3 percent) concluded that there was not" (Hamm et al., 2013).

Social Media and Outreach

Despite the difficulties of measuring social media's use in consumer and patient education, many healthcare groups and organizations are using various social media tools for outreach. A search of the literature revealed that these are primarily hospitals, the government, and nonprofit organizations such as the American Heart Association. Additionally, there are for-profit organizations attempting to use social media to reach consumers. Some are drug companies hoping to advertise their products, and there are patient portals such as PatientsLikeMe, which provide people with a way to share their healthcare experiences.

Ed Bennett created a list of hospitals using social media titled the "Healthcare Social Networking List." The list was hosted on his blog, *Found in Cache*, and was later moved to the Mayo Clinic Center for Social Media, which now maintains it. As of July 2013, more than 1,500 hospitals in the United States are using at least one social media tool (Mayo Clinic, 2012b). Househ found "U.S. healthcare organizations use social media as part of various community engagement activities, such as fundraising, customer service and support, the provision of news and information, patient education and advertising new services" (Househ, 2013, p. 245). Both Househ and the Healthcare Social Networking List cite Facebook as the most-used tool among hospitals. The Healthcare Social Networking List lists 4Square as the second-most-used tool, followed by Twitter, then YouTube. In 2010, the Mayo Clinic established the Social Media Health Network with the mandate, "to accelerate the effective adoption of social media at Mayo Clinic and in healthcare globally" and is "committed to inspiring broader and deeper engagement with social media by hospitals, medical professionals, and patients" (Mayo Clinic, 2012c). Even though many hospitals are using social media, one of the main challenges for institutions is to determine the impact of their social media endeavors. Meaningful use of social media by patients is important to determine its effectiveness as well as to help hospital administrators determine the level of staffing and frequency of updating, promoting, and maintaining their institution's social media presence.

The U.S. government has embraced healthcare social media. The Centers for Disease Control and Prevention (CDC) have an entire website detailing their social media campaigns at http://www.cdc.gov/socialmedia/, and the National Institutes of Health have an inventory of the many social media contacts used by each of its offices and institutes at http://www.nih.gov/ Subscriptions.htm. While hospitals use social media to reach their marketplace's current and potential patients, the government must communicate with the entire U.S. population. The CDC had more than five hundred thousand Facebook fans and over 2.7 million people following on Twitter. Even so, the number of "likes" and "followers" isn't a measure of people's actions, beyond reporting that they once clicked the "like" or "follow" button. As mentioned previously in this chapter, measuring the impact of social media on consumers' actions is difficult. Many of the CDC's Facebook and Twitter posts usually refer to a link or page on the CDC website. By measuring the number of "click-throughs" to CDC.gov content from Facebook and Twitter, site managers are able to get an idea of how many people sought more information. From January 2012 to April 2013, the CDC had anywhere from five thousand to approximately eighteen thousand click-throughs per month from their Facebook posts and approximately four thousand to nine thousand click-throughs per month from their Twitter posts (CDC, 2013). While this doesn't measure what people did with the information from CDC.gov, it does give a snapshot of people's behavior after reading the post.

Many health-related organizations and companies have also expanded into social media as a way to connect to patients. Some of the organizations are not-for-profit groups that have had an established tradition of supporting consumer health information and education. When the American Heart Association released the changes for the 2010 cardiopulmonary resuscitation guidelines, they posted videos on their YouTube channel (http://www .youtube.com/americanheartassoc) demonstrating the "hands only" cardiopulmonary resuscitation. In 2013, the American Heart Association issued a scientific statement on the role of social media for the prevention and management of childhood obesity. "Motivational enhancement delivered through social media (typically facilitated online or through electronic communication by a counselor in a nonjudgmental manner) may be helpful in sustaining efforts in weight loss" (Li et al., 2013, p. 260).

Nonprofit organizations are also partnering with for-profit companies seeking to reach patients. Content communities are good examples of one way organizations partner to provide patients with health information. BBK Worldwide, PatientsLikeMe, and the American Diabetes Association partnered to create the website CallingAllTypes. CallingAllTypes.com "encourages people with Type 1 and Type 2 diabetes to become active members of online health communities such as PatientsLikeMe to help improve and transform the way they manage their own conditions." CallingAllTypes states it will donate one dollar to the American Diabetes Association for each of the first ten thousand unique visitors (CallingAllTypes, 2013). The website seeks to get patients with diabetes to pledge their support and manage their health better. It asks for their email, whether they are a patient with diabetes or caregiver, and asks if they are interested in learning more about medication coverage, clinical studies, resources/tools, and patient communities. BBK Worldwide is a patient recruitment company. PatientsLikeMe is a for-profit company that provides a patient community platform that allows patients to share their experiences and learn from "real-world, outcome based health data" (PatientsLikeMe, 2013). The site is free to join (directly or through CallingAllTypes) and relies on patients to provide personal information about themselves and their diseases or conditions. In return, patients who are living with the same condition are connected and able to learn, communicate, and share with others. As of 2012, PatientsLikeMe had more than 160,000 registered patients and covers more than one thousand diseases. Patients using the PatientsLikeMe platform report high levels of satisfaction, indicating the site made it easier for them to communicate with a support network and make treatment decisions. PatientsLikeMe has "received positive reviews and feedback from other patients, clinicians, and non-profit organizations. Because of this enthusiasm, users have requested the development of a real-world conference that brings together different communities of users" (Agency for Healthcare Research and Quality, 2012).

While a search of the literature revealed several instances of hospital or academic medical libraries using social media for outreach, the majority of these libraries used social media to encourage patrons to use the library, not to provide them with patient education materials or consumer health information. Duhon and Jameson conducted a survey to determine the types of health information outreach activity of approximately 1,700 general academic and academic health sciences libraries. The majority of the respondents (55 percent) indicated their libraries did not conduct consumer health information outreach. Of those libraries engaged, it was primarily to train others to evaluate the quality of consumer health information and also to publicize resources via a blog or website. More than three-quarters of all respondents "perceived at least some need for HIO [health information outreach] at their library, while under half were actually fulfilling that need by delivering HIO" (Duhon and Jameson, 2013). Duhon and Jameson found these results to be very similar to those of other studies that mention a "gap between what libraries perceive they need to do, and what they are actually doing to administer HIO" (Duhon and Jameson, 2013). Duhon and Jameson did not specifically study the use of social media for consumer health information outreach; only one question on the survey mentioned the use of social media (blogs). However, if the majority are not conducting outreach at all, then even fewer are using social media to provide consumer health information.

Bright Lights: Aurora Health Care System libraries developed a new consumer health service for their organization in 2006, and the service has evolved over time to include using social media to deliver consumer health information. The Aurora Libraries' Facebook page is targeted to consumers (Donahue et al., 2012). As of July 2013, it had 431 people who "like" the page (Aurora Health Care Libraries, 2013). Librarians and library assistants post links on the Facebook page to current health issues research or consumer book reviews. Nutritional and emotional health posts are the most popular items on the page (Donahue et al., 2012).

Even though the library literature has little on the use of social media to provide consumer health information and patient education, a discussion of medical librarians on Twitter revealed some librarians are engaged in this work (Social Media, 2013). One of the libraries mentioned in the discussion was the University of Michigan Taubman Health Sciences Library, which has both a Twitter feed (@MLibraryHealthy) and Facebook page (https://www.facebook.com/MlibraryHealthy) dedicated to providing consumer health information. As of July 2013, this library has 1,523 Twitter followers and posted 10,130 tweets, the majority of which are dedicated to consumer and public health information (Taubman Twitter, 2013).

The MLibrary Health Communities were also created as an effort to provide different methods of consumer health outreach by the Coordinator of Outreach Services and Liaison Librarian at the University of Michigan Taubman Health Sciences Library. According to Saylor, both sites evolved into successful methods of providing consumer health information outreach. Unfortunately, it became more difficult to judge whether posts were reaching their intended audience because Facebook changed its software and usage metrics (Saylor, 2013). Their Facebook page has 629 "likes" with posts also dedicated to consumer health information (Taubman Facebook, 2013).

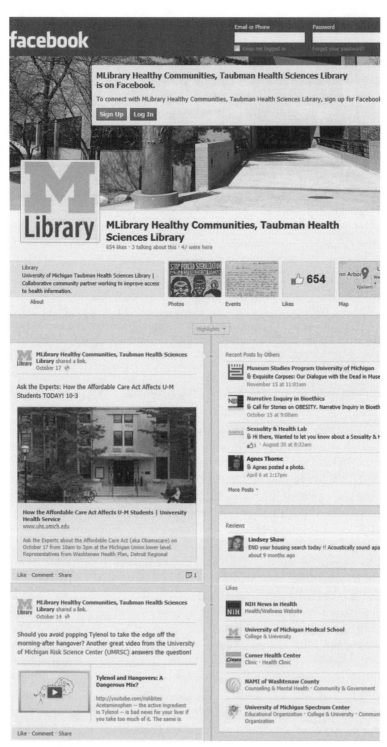

FIGURE 9.4
Screen Shot of the MLibrary Healthy Community Facebook Page, University of Michigan Taubman Health Sciences Library Collaborative

Also mentioned during the social media discussion on Twitter was the University of Massachusetts Medical School Lamar Soutter Library Women's Health LibGuide project. The Women's LibGuide project was made possible by a National Library of Medicine and National Institutes of Health grant. "The overall aim of the project is to improve and promote access to women's health resources within UMMS, specifically among faculty engaged in research in this area, as well as the students and residents they teach" (Moyer, 2013). A LibGuide was created featuring women's health research and local resources. The library's Twitter account (@UMMSLibrary) was used to promote the women's health resources on the LibGuide. The LibGuide had 1,602 views since launching its social media campaign on Twitter on May 17, 2013, and resulted in a 65 percent increase in followers in one week. Within one month, the Women's Health Outreach LibGuide appeared in the Lamar Soutter Library's Top Ten LibGuide Rankings. While a qualitative assessment is still under way to determine the scope of its success, the library has already submitted a request for continued funding, and plans are under way to develop another grant proposal to expand the project (Moyer, 2013). Lamar Soutter Library's program closely resembles the CDC's approach to connecting consumer health information social media outreach to their websites, providing more in-depth information.

Creating a Social Media Presence for Libraries

"Social media tools should not be taken lightly or applied blindly. The keys to a successful strategy are planning collaboratively and applying the right technology to the right need for the right users" (Thielst, 2010, p. 64). Should a library want to use social media to provide consumer health and patient information, there are several factors to consider. It is important to create a social media plan ahead of time. The plan should include technology needed, support or approval from the institution, tool selection, effectiveness measures, and risks, concerns, and barriers and how to overcome them. The social media plan, once implemented, should be reevaluated periodically. "Correctly applied, social media tools will build trust and loyalty among stake holders" (Thielst, 2010, p. 64). Trust and loyalty are especially important when providing consumer health and patient information.

Technology and Institutional Support

It is essential to have the support or approval of the institution prior to engaging in social media on behalf of the library. Some hospitals have restrictions as to what social media products may be accessed within the institution. Many institutions have strong control over their brand, the use of their name, and representation; therefore, they have regulations as to who can deploy social media on behalf of the institution. The Mayo Clinic's social media guidelines for its employees outline specifically how employees should represent and conduct themselves. These guidelines state employees should not have a social media name or "handle," and no personal URL should include Mayo Clinic's name or logo (Mayo Clinic, 2012a). The Aurora Libraries worked with the Aurora Health Care social media department, enabling them to send posts about their library and consumer health information through the institution's Aurora Health Care Twitter feed and Facebook page (Donahue et al., 2012, p. 63).

Librarians interested in consumer and patient health information outreach via social media might consider partnering with a local public library. The literature contains many examples of medical and public libraries collaborating to provide consumer health information. Cushing/Whitney Medical Library, Hill Regional Career High School, the New Haven Free Public Library, and Yale University's Office of New Haven and State Affairs partnered on a National Network of Libraries of Medicine outreach project targeting health information literacy among urban teens through the creation of web videos on YouTube (Greenberg and Wang, 2012, p. 135). While social media itself was not the reason these institutions collaborated, such partnerships with outside entities may afford librarians an avenue to use social media while still following hospital policy.

Focus and Selection of Tools

The CDC's social media toolkit states, "the keys to effective social media outreach are identifying target audience(s), determining objective(s), knowing outlet(s) and deciding on the amount of resources (time and effort) that can be invested" (CDC, 2011, p. 5). Determining the target audience is extremely important. There are thousands of diseases, conditions, and consumer health topics, so trying to cover them all would lead to fragmentation and loss of focus. The site PatientsLikeMe, which now covers more than one thousand disease topics, began with just one disease, amyotrophic lateral sclerosis (Agency for Healthcare Research and Quality, 2012). Target audiences can be as broad as women's health or as narrow as those suffering from a specific malady such as stroke. A library's social media project may be intended for a specific audience, but librarians may discover others are interested as well. Upon reviewing the followers of the MLibrary Healthy Twitter and Facebook projects, Saylor noted that in addition to consumers following the MLibrary Healthy accounts, other entities such as libraries, government organizations, nonprofit organizations, etc., were also followers. As a result, posts were expanded to include more library and general medical information and news (Saylor, 2013).

Once a target audience or subject has been selected, clarifying the objective is necessary as it will be a factor in selecting usage and measurement tools. "Measurable objectives are the key to successful evaluation and ultimately successful programs" (Whitney, Dutcher, and Kesleman, 2013, p. 142). If the objective is to simply distribute information for consumers to view, then selecting a tool(s) that measures likes, re-tweets, or views may be all that is necessary. Some measurement tools reside within the platform, such as Facebook, while others come from third-party companies that monitor social media sites, such as Twitter. While convenient, these tools tend to change their measurement parameters quite often and sometimes have vague methodologies for scores. Saylor expressed frustration with Facebook's changes in its usage statistics platform, noting the documentation was lacking and modifications in its algorithm made it difficult to compare usage over time (Saylor, 2013). The more complex the objective, the more complicated the tools or procedures needed to measure its effectiveness. For example, if the objective is to use social media to provide health information to improve consumers' health behavior or overall health, then the librarian needs to plan to select appropriate tools or evaluation methods for measuring those objectives. "The greatest challenge of health information outreach is the gap between what researchers would like to measure and what can be realistically measured" (Whitney, Dutcher, and Kesleman, 2013, p. 139).

As mentioned previously, selecting a social media tool is predicated upon defining the audience and objective. Doing so helps the librarian determine whether to use a collaborative project tool, blog or microblog, content community, social networking site, or virtual gaming or social world. Fortunately, librarians are not limited to just one type of tool and may select more than one. Many of these tools work with each other, making it easier to propagate the message or content across multiple platforms. For example, a librarian can post within Facebook and have those posts show up as tweets in their Twitter accounts. Not only do hospitals do this between Facebook and Twitter but they often include a link to their website, thus driving consumers to a page providing more information than just a short paragraph on Facebook or a 140 character message. As mentioned earlier, the CDC measures the number of "click-throughs" to their CDC.gov content from Facebook and Twitter, providing them with the number of people who sought more information on a topic or tweet.

Even though social media tools often work with each other, creating and maintaining a social media presence requires librarians' time and effort.

Deciding frequency of updates and information is critical. Nothing is more frustrating that seeing an interesting social media site only to learn it hasn't been updated in years. Blogs are notorious for this, begun for a particular reason but left forgotten and unrevised as the author has ceased posting. The Internet can be a graveyard to social media projects left abandoned. It is necessary to decide who will contribute, review, and post content. While multiple people can contribute content, it is usually best to limit the number of people involved in order to minimize confusion and provide a singular voice. It is important to ensure those responsible for the social media outreach have the time and skills to continually develop and maintain the project. In their You-Tube project, Greenberg and Wang described the challenges with recruiting and retaining the student video mentor who maintained project timelines, goals, and reporting guidelines (Greenberg and Wang, 2012). Changes may occur where the person dedicated to the project can no longer maintain the social media presence. This could be due to a change in the person's other job duties or because the project has grown significantly since its inception. As a result, other persons may need to be added to the project or the amount of time devoted to keep the project going may need to be revised. Likewise, finding the right staff and scheduling proper time can have a positive effect on the project. Saylor noted the MLibrary Healthy Twitter account flourished when the outreach assistant responsible for maintaining the account, a student from the School of Public Health: Health Behavior & Health Education, became especially active and engaged in the project (Saylor, 2013).

Risks and Concerns of Social Media Outreach

Unfortunately, the use of social media carries certain risk and concerns, thus providing health information via social media does, too. The protection of one's privacy is extremely important. The very participatory nature and openness of communicating through social media makes it even more important that HIPAA compliancy be maintained. Because each social media tool operates differently and people share diverse types of information, it is necessary to adapt precautions to fit each social media tool. For example, the precautions one would take for Twitter may be different from those one would apply to the medical image sharing application as shown in the Figure 1 screen shot.

The sharing nature of social media means that information has the potential to reach millions of people. Librarians are usually very good at vetting health information resources, but one needs to be mindful that users may share unverified information. This happens often on sites like Facebook and other community platforms. Greene analyzed diabetic communities within Facebook and discovered a variety of participants on the sites. Patients, caregivers, advertisers, and researchers with different perspectives and motivations would post health and disease management information "not necessarily available through more formal channels of professional consultation" (Greene et al., 2011, p. 291). This can make it difficult for moderators and consumers alike to know what information they can trust. The "inability to verify the identity of the poster and prominent use of Facebook pages for the promotion of non-FDA-approved therapeutic modalities poses a significant problem to the trustworthiness of any single piece of information on this widely used online social networking tool" (Greene et al., 2011, p. 291). The risks associated with social media should not dissuade users; however, these risks must be considered and addressed.

Conclusion

Usage of social media continues to grow. The percentage of users on Twitter has doubled since November 2010, and nearly two-thirds of online adult users claim to be Facebook users. Pinterest has garnered 15 percent of Internet users, and 13 percent of Internet users are on Instagram. While social media are primarily used by those younger than fifty years old, it has crossed ethnic lines. Seventy-two percent of Hispanic and sixty-eight percent of black non-Hispanic Internet users are on social media (Duggan and Brenner, 2013). Social media is an online communication network used in U.S. presidential elections, to drive social change, and provide information in times of disasters. It can be leveraged to extend current consumer and patient health information outreach beyond a one-on-one, face-to-face model. It has the ability to reach many more users than any one person can do physically. Today's librarians must create a social media plan that clearly defines goals and methods to achieve them, yet is flexible enough to deal with the constantly changing landscape of social media and users. It is also crucial that librarians appropriately measure their efforts. "One of the main challenges for healthcare organizations is related to understanding the meaningful use of social media sites by patients. Merely visiting a Facebook page or viewing a YouTube video doe not signify meaningful use" (Househ, 2013, p. 245). New methods of social media measurement will help librarians justify its expense in money, time, and personnel to the library's administration. The popularity of the tools and the ability to reach multiple people makes social media for community and patient health information an interesting and possibly successful method to extend the library's outreach.

References

Agency for Healthcare Research and Quality. 2012. "Online Communities Foster Data Sharing, Communication, and Learning among Patients with Neurologic and Other Chronic Diseases." *AHRQ Health Care Innovations Exchange*, Service Delivery Innovation Profile, October 10, 2012. http://www.innovations.ahrq.gov/content.aspx?id=1801. Accessed June 19, 2013.

American Cancer Society. 2012. "History of RFL of SL." Relay for Life. http://rflofsl.intuitwebsites.com/History-of-RFL-of-SL.html. Accessed July 8, 2013.

Aurora Health Care Libraries. 2013. Facebook Page. https://www.facebook.com/auroralibraries. Accessed July 12, 2013.

Beaumont, P. 2011. "The Truth about Twitter, Facebook and the Uprisings in the Arab World." *The Guardian*. February 24, 2011. http://www.guardian.co.uk/world/2011/feb/25/twitter-facebook-uprisings-arab-libya. Accessed June 19, 2013.

Blackwell, T. 2013. "New Medical Photo-Sharing App not for the Faint of Heart as Doctors Upload Strange, Gruesome Images." *National Post*. June 9, 2013. http://news.nationalpost.com/2013/06/09/figure1-app-not-for-the-faint-of-heart-as-doctors-upload-gruesome-images/. Accessed July 5, 2013.

Boulos, MN, Hetherington, L, and Wheeler, S. 2007. "Second Life: An Overview of the Potential of 3-D Virtual Worlds in Medical and Health Education." *Health Information and Libraries Journal*, 24:233.

Bow, HD, et al., 2013. "A Crowdsourcing Model for Creating Preclinical Medical Education Study Tools." *Academic Medicine*, 88:766.

Bronk, C, and Smith, T. 2010. "Diplopedia Imagined: Building State's Diplomacy Wiki." Preconference draft at the 2010 International Symposium on Collaborative Technologies and Systems, Chicago, IL, May 17–21, 2010. http://www.bakerinstitute.org/publications/TSPP-pub-BronkSmithDiplopediaDraft-051810.pdf. Accessed July 1, 2013.

Buie, A, and Smith Jones, M. 2011. "Responding to Healthcare Consumerism with Social Media: How Social Media and Collaborative Tools Are Transforming Healthcare Delivery." *Preficient Healthcare White Paper*. September 2011. http://www.perficient.com/Thought-Leadership/White-Papers/2011/Healthcare-Consumerism-and-Social-Media. Accessed July 8, 2013.

CallingAllTypes. 2013. "CallingAllTypes FAQs." http://www.callingalltypes.com/faqs.html. Accessed June 19, 2013.

Cave, D. 2011. "Mexico Turns to Social Media for Information and Survival." *New York Times*. September 24, 2011. http://www.nytimes.com/2011/09/25/world/americas/mexico-turns-to-twitter-and-facebook-for-information-and-survival.html. Accessed June 19, 2013.

Centers for Disease Control and Prevention. 2011. "The Health Communicator's Social Media Toolkit." July 2011. http://www.cdc.gov/socialmedia/tools/guidelines/pdf/socialmediatoolkit_bm.pdf. Accessed July 12, 2013.

Centers for Disease Control and Prevention. 2013. "CDC.gov and Social Media Metrics: April 2013." CDC Metrics Dashboard, April 2013. http://www.cdc.gov/metrics/reports/2013/oadcmetricsreportapril2013.pdf. Accessed July 10, 2013.

Cohen, SE. 2013. "Sandy Marked a Shift for Social Media Use in Disasters." *Emergency Management*. March 7, 2013. http://www.emergencymgmt.com/disaster/Sandy -Social-Media-Use-in-Disasters.html. Accessed June 24, 2013.

Donahue, A, et al. 2012. "Consumer Health Outreach as a Sum of Parts: Individual and Collective Approaches of a Health Care System's Libraries." *Journal of Hospital Librarianship*, 12:61.

Duggan, M, and Brenner, J. 2013. "The Demographics of Social Media Users—2012." Pew Research Center's Internet & American Life Project, February 14, 2013. http:// pewinternet.org/Reports/2013/Social-media-users.aspx. Accessed July 8, 2013.

Duhon, L, and Jameson, J. 2013. "Health Information Outreach: A Survey of U.S. Academic Libraries, Highlighting a Midwestern University's Experience." *Health Information and Libraries Journal*, 30:121.

Gray, P. 2013. "Second Life Celebrates 10-Year Anniversary." *Linden Lab Press Release*. June 20, 2013. http://lindenlab.com/releases/second-life-celebrates-10-year -anniversary. Accessed July 8, 2013.

Greenberg, CJ, and Wang, L. 2012. "Building Health Literacy among an Urban Teenage Population by Creating Online Health Videos for Public and School Health Curriculum Use." *Journal of Consumer Health on the Internet*, 16:135.

Greene, JA, et al. 2011. "Online Social Networking by Patients with Diabetes: A Qualitative Evaluation of Communication with Facebook." *Journal of General Internal Medicine*, 26:287–92.

Hamm, MP, et al. 2013. "Social Media Use among Patients and Caregivers: A Scoping Review." *BMJ Open*, 3:1–9.

Hardenbrook, J. 2011. "I Graduated from a Top Library School. Yeah, So What?" *Mr. Library Dude*. July 1, 2011. http://mrlibrarydude.wordpress.com/2011/07/21/ i-graduated-from-a-top-library-school-yeah-so-what/. Accessed July 5, 2013.

Homeland Security. 2013. "Lessons Learned: Social Media and Hurricane Sandy." U.S. Department of Homeland Security. Science and Technology Directorate. Virtual Social Media Working Group and DHS First Responders Group. June 2013. https:// communities.firstresponder.gov/DHS_VSMWG_Lessons_Learned_Social_Media_ and_Hurricane_Sandy_Formatted_June_2013_FINAL.pdf. Accessed June 23, 2013.

Househ, M. 2013. "The Use of Social Media in Healthcare: Organizational, Clinical, and Patient Perspectives." *Studies in Health Technologies and Informatics*, 183:244–48.

Jones, C. 2012. "Olympics 2012: Twitter Users Blamed for Disrupting BBC's Cycling Coverage." *The Guardian*. July 29, 2012. http://www.guardian.co.uk/media/2012/ jul/29/olympics-2012-twitter-bbc-cycling. Accessed June 18, 2013.

Kennel, K, Collazo-Clavell, ML, and Richards, ML. 2013. "16th Annual Mayo Clinic Endocrine Course." Mayo School of Continuous Professional Development. February 2, 2013. http://www.mayo.edu/cme/endocrinology-2013r170/section ID/D1FB1150-22C5-11E2-AA810050569C0CB4/subsectionID/9A854370-22C6 -11E2-AA810050569C0CB4. Accessed July 8, 2013.

Laird, S. 2012. "World's First Live-Tweeted Open Heart Surgery Is a Success [PICS]." Mashable. February 23, 2012. http://mashable.com/2012/02/23/tweeted-open -heart-surgery/. Accessed June 15, 2013.

Li, JS, et al. 2013. "Approaches to the Prevention and Management of Childhood Obesity: The Role of Social Networks and the Use of Social Media and Related Electronic Technologies: A Scientific Statement from the American Heart Association." *Circulation*, 127:260.

Lunden, I. 2012. "Analyst: Twitter Passed 500M Users in June 2012, 140M of Them in US; Jakarta 'Biggest Tweeting' City." TechCrunch. July 30, 2012. http://tech crunch.com/2012/07/30/analyst-twitter-passed-500m-users-in-june-2012-140m -of-them-in-us-jakarta-biggest-tweeting-city/. Accessed July 5, 2013.

Mayo Clinic. 2012a. "For Mayo Clinic Employees." *Sharing Mayo Clinic*. http://shar ing.mayoclinic.org/guidelines/for-mayo-clinic-employees/. Accessed July 12, 2013.

Mayo Clinic. 2012b. "Hospital Social Networking List." Social Media Health Network. http://network.socialmedia.mayoclinic.org/hcsml-grid/. Accessed July 9, 2013.

Mayo Clinic. 2012c. "Introducing the Hospital Social Networking List." Social Media Health Network. September 12, 2012. http://network.socialmedia.mayoclinic .org/2012/09/12/introducing-the-health-care-social-media-list/. Accessed July 9, 2013.

Moyer, J. 2013. Email program overview message to author, July 17, 2013.

Ovide, S. 2012. "Twitter Embraces Olympics to Train for the Big Time." *Wall Street Journal*. July 23, 2012. http://on.wsj.com/NqOfyG. Accessed June 18, 2013.

PatientsLikeMe. 2013. "PatientsLikeMe About Us." http://www.patientslikeme.com/ about. Accessed June 19, 2013.

Saylor, K. 2013. In discussion with author, July 16, 2013.

Social Media. 2013. #Medlibs Chat Transcript. July 11, 2013. http://bit.ly/1b4Xv6C. Accessed July 12, 2013.

Tam, D. 2013. "Facebook by the Numbers: 1.06 Billion Monthly Active Users." *CNET News*. January 30, 2013. http://news.cnet.com/8301-1023_3-57566550-93/face book-by-the-numbers-1.06-billion-monthly-active-users/. Accessed July 5, 2013.

Taubman Facebook. 2013. Taubman Health Sciences Library MLibrary Healthy Communities Facebook Page. https://www.facebook.com/MlibraryHealthy. Accessed July 12, 2013.

Taubman Twitter. 2013. Taubman Health Sciences Library @MLibraryHealthy Twitter Page. https://twitter.com/MLibraryHealthy. Accessed July 12, 2013.

Thielst, CB. 2010. *Social Media in Healthcare*. Chicago: Health Administration Press.

U.S. National Library of Medicine/Greater Midwest Region. 2006. "Consumer Health Subcontract Recipients." http://nnlm.gov/gmr/funding/consumer/recipients.html. Accessed July 8, 2013.

Whitney, W, Dutcher, GA, and Kesleman, A. 2013. "Evaluation of Health Information Outreach: Theory, Practice, and Future Direction." *Journal of the Medical Library Association*, 10:138–46.

Zachte, E. 2012. "Wikimedia Report Card February 2012." *Wikipedia*. April 2012. http://stats.wikimedia.org/reportcard/. Accessed July 1, 2013.

10

Meeting the Needs of Diverse Groups: Children, Teens, LGBT, and Patients with Low Literacy

Linda Stahl

MEETING THE UNIQUE AND DIVERSE health information needs of the people consumer health librarians serve can be a daunting challenge. It requires an awareness of community to develop an appropriate collection and the myriad resources required. Each day brings requests and questions from people varying in age, race, ethnic backgrounds, sexual orientation, and physical and mental abilities. To provide the best service in an appropriate format for their clients, librarians must call upon their deep knowledge of health information resources and have a solid understanding of age-based needs, cultural awareness, and sensitivity. The constantly changing technology landscape is challenging for staff to keep up with, yet it is vital considering today's adolescents have grown up in the age of Internet, social media, and cell phone technology. Locating credible and reliable health information to answer their questions requires knowledge of how to evaluate and sift through the vast amount of information online. On the other hand, many older adults, patrons with limited English, and persons with low-literacy skills are often not computer literate and require the expertise of a librarian to help them access online resources. Lesbian, gay, bisexual, and transgender (LGBT) equality has made great strides in the last decade, but LGBT individuals continue to face discrimination in many areas including access to health. Creating a safe and welcoming space to meet the information needs of the most vulnerable in our communities is a critical mission of the consumer health library. The ability to meet people on their terms increases the likelihood of providing them with suitable health information thus helping each to be better informed healthcare consumers, work as partners with their healthcare providers, and better able to manage their own health. This begins with treating everyone encountered, whether in person or online, with the respect and compassion they deserve.

The ability to create that safe and welcoming space begins with each individual. Librarians come to work each day with their own set of beliefs, values, knowledge, and life experience. This can shape the way librarians react to and interact with patients and consumers. Chapter 11 thoroughly examines the issue of cultural sensitivity in relation to the provision of health information, but there are some basic assumptions around cultural competency that are worthy of reflection and mentioning when serving diverse populations (Purnell and Paulanka, 2008). The following tips can be used universally with each interaction:

- One culture is not better than another culture, just different.
- Culture has a powerful influence on one's interpretation of and responses to healthcare.
- Each individual has a right to be respected for his or her uniqueness and/ or cultural heritage.
- Prejudices and biases can be minimized with cultural understanding.
- Every client encounter is a cultural encounter.

Each person interacted with carries within them influences of gender, family, friends, religion, community, education, and a myriad of other factors, including the concerns that brought them through the door to the library. Healthcare delivery is changing rapidly and continues to evolve. There is the expectation in healthcare today that individuals and patients play a larger role than ever before in managing their health. Yet inequalities and challenges to access to care remain for many. Consumer health librarians can help reduce some of these disparities by meeting the challenge of offering health information resources to diverse communities. Welcoming all with compassion and a sincere desire to help will create a comfortable space for people to find answers to their questions surrounding disease, treatment, recovery, and wellness.

Reference Interview for Special Populations

The consumer health reference interview is one of the best skills a librarian can perfect in the provision of health information. It's assumed that in many, if not most, cases, patrons have already done a bit of research before they enter the library. Regardless of whether they consulted a friend, relative, healthcare provider, book, or the Internet, the library is often at the end of the list for people searching for health information. In the meantime, the information they've retrieved may be of poor quality, incomplete, or inaccurate.

As outlined in Chapter 7, the basis of any health reference interview is to ask open-ended questions: who, what, when, where, how, and why. This approach helps to clarify the person's health question along with what sites or resources he or she has already looked at before turning to the library. Consumer health questions run the gamut from the mundane to a life and death health crisis to a sensitive or stigmatizing issue around sexuality or mental health. The individual may feel scared, embarrassed, or uncertain about how to approach and even ask for assistance. While, detailed information about conducting the health reference interview is found in Chapter 7 of this book, the following points are essential and bear repeating when conducting any interview:

- Be clear that the consumer/patient can count on confidentiality.
- Make sure the nature of the question is understood.
- Provide some privacy, especially if the question is of a sensitive nature.

An inviting physical environment plays a large role in making people feel welcome and comfortable. From the signage on doors and walls, to brochures and materials within the collection of the consumer health library, users notice and pick up on these clues and cues:

- Display pictures and posters reflecting the diversity within your community.
- Identify bilingual staff members.
- Provide health information brochures in the languages that reflect the various cultures within your community.

Meeting the Needs of Children

Health information for children under the age of twelve is most often needed by parents to help their child understand a condition or diagnosis. It may be a diagnosis the child is facing, or to help them cope with the illness of a parent, sibling, or grandparent. Health collections should include a variety of age-appropriate books, DVDs, and multimedia models that can be used to support parents in their role as caregivers and to assist them in their role of being part of their child's healthcare team. These materials also help children understand more about their own health condition or that of their family member.

Providing contact information for local or regional support groups and national organizations and websites, including those with interactive games, videos, and tutorials especially for children, will be welcome resources for children and families.

Apart from age-appropriate children's health information resources, include a "children's corner" in your library with puzzles, books depicting the diverse populations and languages in your community, and other toys that can help occupy children, thus giving parents and caregivers precious time to focus on getting their own health information.

Today's consumer health libraries are providing creative and innovative opportunities to disseminate health information to children to help them learn and begin to form healthy habits that will last a lifetime. Promising programs link consumer health librarians with natural partners and resources in the community. Consider developing a Healthy Summer Story Time in partnership with a local public library with a focus on teaching children, through stories and activities, about nutrition, exercise and activity, safety, illness prevention, and stress reduction. Such programs offer a way to introduce parents to the consumer health library. The program may also provide opportunities to partner with other local groups serving children including schools, migrant programs, and even local public health departments and clinics. This is an ideal, entertaining way to offer age-appropriate information while building children's health, wellness, and prevention skills. Bilingual library staff or community partners are integral to reaching out and connecting with local organizations serving children whose primary language is not English.

Strategies for a successful interaction include the following:

- When body language suggests worry or apprehension, smile, stand, and approach them with a warm greeting.
- Stoop to greet the child and include him or her in the interaction.
- Use open-ended questions to determine the information, quality, and source (e.g., books, online or mobile apps, or videos) the parent has already reviewed.
- Ask what the parent would most like to know (e.g., treatment, tests, procedures, or comfort measures, etc.). Focus on the "need to know" information to avoid overwhelming the parent with too much information.
- Explain the different types and technical level of information available along with the variety of formats. Allow the patron to choose what she is most comfortable with.
- Remember to include the child by offering age-appropriate information from the bookshelves or interactive website that can help the child understand his or her newly diagnosed condition.
- Check back to ask if the parent needs more assistance.

TABLE 10.1
Snapshot of Strategies in Action:
Successful Interaction for Children's Health Information

A young mother with her eight-year-old daughter stepped into the Resource Center and glanced around with an uncertain look on her face. Ruth, the reference librarian, looked up from her desk, smiled, and walked over to where the mother and daughter stood. "Welcome, how may I help you?" Ruth asked.

"I was told I could find some information about childhood asthma here," the mother responded. "My daughter, Ella, was in the hospital for three days last week. I thought she had a bad chest cold, but then one night she just couldn't catch her breath, we were all so scared—we ended up in the ER. The discharge nurse suggested I come here to get information about asthma before our follow-up appointment with Ella's doctor. And, do you have something that might help Ella understand what asthma is so she won't be so scared if she gets sick again?"

Ruth bent down and said to Ella, "I'm really glad you're feeling better, Ella. I think we have some information that will help you and your mom learn more about asthma. Can you tell me how old you are? Eight—that's great!" Ruth stood and asked Ella's mom, "What are you most interested in knowing about asthma before the follow-up appointment?"

"Everything, but they mentioned 'asthma triggers' and 'rescue medication' in the hospital. It sounds like lots of things can cause an asthma attack. We have a dog. I'd like to know more about that," said the mom.

"Okay," said Ruth. "We have some excellent resources on asthma in children that will explain what asthma is, including asthma triggers and the different medicines used to treat it. I can show you some books and excellent websites for both parents and kids with asthma in Ella's age group. Where would you like to start?"

Ella's mom smiled and relaxed a bit, "I'd like to see the books first."

TABLE 10.2
Children's Health Resources

American Academy of Pediatrics
http://www.healthychildren.org
  The American Academy of Pediatrics provides this parent-/consumer-oriented website with information on a variety of topics from infant and child development, safety and prevention, health issues, and more.

Kids Eat Right
http://www.eatright.org/kids/
  The Academy of Nutrition and Dietetics created the Kids Eat Right website specifically for child nutrition from infancy through adolescence with access to articles, recipes, videos, and more. Up to date and scientifically supported.

(continued)

TABLE 10.2
(continued)

Kids Health
http://kidshealth.org/
   From the Nemours Foundation, a nonprofit organization dedicated to children's health, Kids Health provides information about children's health, behavior, and development from before birth through the teen years. There are separate sections for kids, teens, and parents.

Medical Library Association Consumer and Patient Health Information Section (CAPHIS)
http://caphis.mlanet.org/consumer/parenting13.html
   CAPHIS lists its recommended websites and resources on children's health and parenting based upon their criteria for evaluating information on the Internet.

MedlinePlus Children's Health Page
http://www.nlm.nih.gov/medlineplus/childrenshealth.html
   This link is one of several from the National Library of Medicine's MedlinePlus website that deals with children and child development.

Nutrition Websites for Kids and Teens
http://kingcounty.gov/healthservices/health/nutrition/schools/youth.aspx
   King County Public Health offers links to interactive tools helping kids of all ages learn about nutrition and health.

We Can!
http://www.nhlbi.nih.gov/health/public/heart/obesity/wecan/
   We Can! from the National Health Lung and Blood Institute is a website devoted to helping parents and families develop healthy eating habits and get active through fun activities and reducing screen time.

Meeting the Needs of Teens and Adolescents

When it comes to providing health information, teens and adolescents can pose some particular and specific challenges. First, this is a generally healthy demographic and second, it is a stage of life when privacy, confidentiality, and trust are essential. Developmentally, they are experiencing rapid physical, emotional, cognitive, and social change (Smart et al., 2012). Then there is the issue of technology and the role it plays in the lives of adolescents. This generation has grown up in the age of social media and smart phones. Trying to keep up with technological advances with limited time and staff is a very real issue for librarians in general, but it is crucial, as all age groups in our society use the Internet for every kind of information, especially health information.

   The majority of U.S. teenagers aged twelve to seventeen are online (93 percent), and they are using the Internet to seek health information (Borzekowski et al., 2012). The use of technology for these "digital natives" moves across socioeconomic, race, and cultural barriers. They have never lived without pervasive technology in their lives; never known a time without smartphones, Facebook, or Twitter. A new term, "eHealth," encompasses the widespread use of Internet searches to obtain health information; a related term, "eHealth literacy," recognizes the skills needed to ensure such information is derived from sound medical practice. eHealth literacy is a combination of eHealth and health literacy, and defined as "the use of emerging information and communication technology, especially the Internet, to improve or enable health and health care" (Paek and Hove, 2012).

These skills are the same skills librarians use and teach day in and day out: the ability to evaluate, use, and apply health information to users' personal lives. There is an enormous opportunity for librarians to have a positive impact on the health of teens as they age. Low health literacy is known to be associated with risky health behaviors in teens. While this group on the whole is healthy, their greatest threats are substance abuse (including tobacco), sexually transmitted infections, and teen pregnancy. Other areas of health concern that teens and adolescents have identified include:

- Anxiety.
- Depression and mental health issues including stress.
- Specific illness (e.g., cancer, diabetes, asthma).
- Nutrition, especially related to sports performance.
- Sleep issues.

Helping teens and adolescents learn to evaluate traditional and eHealth resources for credible and reliable information offers librarians a role in developing a generation with the skills needed to navigate all the avenues of information open to them. This may in turn produce young adults who are health-literate consumers better equipped to manage their well-being as they age, and thereby reduce poor health outcomes for future generations.

One way to accomplish this goal of developing health literate youth is working with local middle and high school health classes. Successful programs that teach teens to be smart health information consumers begin by reaching out to health teachers and school librarians to discuss the value of the consumer health library for their students. Together with instructors, consumer health librarians can develop programs that introduce adolescent users to the consumer health library in a way that is instructive, interactive, and achieves the goal of teaching lifelong health literacy skills and promoting health-seeking behaviors in these digital natives.

Like their adult counterparts, teenagers vary in the way they like to receive health information. When actively seeking health information through a face-to-face encounter, trust is of utmost importance. They are not likely

Bright Lights: Planetree Health Resource Center staff in The Dalles, Oregon, work with health classes in a rural school district. Students begin with a tour of the consumer health library, then the librarian reviews the basics of evaluating and sorting through health information including currency, authorship or evidence, bias, quality, and source (.gov, .edu, .com, .net, etc.) of websites. The students are introduced to MedlinePlus from the National Library of Medicine. They learn how to navigate the different areas of the MedlinePlus website to look up health information including health topics, drug information, and videos and tools. An exercise follows in which the students then select from a basket predetermined, disease-specific topics as well as topics that are of special interest to adolescents. The students must then research the topic they draw from the basket using at least three credible, evidence-based resources from the consumer health library. One of the sources must come from MedlinePlus. Using the resources they find, they write a two-page paper citing sources about the selected topic, which is then shared in class. Teachers and students are very positive about the program, and library staff report students returning to the consumer health library, often with a parent, friend, or other family member.

to approach any individual they feel will judge them negatively, especially if their information request is of a sensitive nature. Use plain language free of library jargon and acronyms. Don't assume they understand the meaning of "monograph" or "periodical." Explain terms and meanings. Children's and teens' vocabulary is still developing, so ask for clarification if there is confusion about pronunciation. Be respectful and treat their questions as seriously as you would an adult. Emphasize that all health questions and information requests are private. As with any library user, offer information in a variety of formats—books, magazines, websites—and allow the adolescent to select what best suits his or her preference for receiving information.

Strategies for a successful interaction include the following:

- Approach teenagers with open body language and a smile.
- Speak in a non-judgmental and respectful tone.
- Step to a more private area away from other library users.
- Be sure to face the teen as you are speaking and maintain eye contact. Have a compassionate and professional attitude and emphasize that every conversation is confidential.
- Offer a variety of resources at varying levels of literacy and allow the teen to select what is appropriate. Include professional hotline and online and local support.
- Tell the teen you'll check back in a few minutes in case he or she has any other questions.

TABLE 10.3
Snapshot of Strategies in Action: Successful Interaction for Teen Health Information

Jenny had been at the reference desk for a while when she thought she'd make a sweep through the library to check on patrons who might need further help. She noticed a teenaged boy who she'd seen earlier at the computer stations. He was browsing the shelves looking a bit lost. Jenny walked over to him with a warm smile, "Hi, my name is Jenny. What may I help you find?" she asked.

The boy smiled shyly and replied in a low voice, "Well, umm, I don't know if you have anything, but I want to find information on supplements for athletes," he said.

"OK, are you an athlete, or is this for a report?" asked Jenny.

The boy responded, "Well, both actually. I play baseball, but I have to do a report for my health class."

"I see," said Jenny. "What type of supplements do you want to find out about?"

"I don't know, anything that can help improve my game," he shrugged. "I've read a couple of articles in some sports magazines, and now it's all over the news about guys using drugs to play better ball. I mean, what's the big deal? I'd like to get a scholarship to play college ball and it's super competitive out there. I'm pretty good, and who knows, I might even go pro if I'm good enough."

"Well, I see you're smart, too, with your decision to research more about this topic here. Supplements and steroids can have a lot of serious side effects, and some are legal and others aren't. I can show you some reliable resources that can answer your questions about the safety and legal issues around performance-enhancing drugs and supplements," Jenny replied. "And I'd like to show you a website called MedlinePlus from the National Library of Medicine. Have you heard of it before?"

"No, I haven't. I've searched Google and a lot of the things that come up want to sell me something. I really want to know what they do that's so dangerous," he responded.

"Well," Jenny said, "there are resources that can help to answer these questions. I'll share some tips that can help you know what to look for when evaluating the good, the bad, and the ugly of online information. You mentioned you are doing a report for your health class. What other types of resources would you like to look at?" Jenny asked as she led him over to a computer station. "I have some books on sports performance and nutrition, would you like to see those as well?"

"Sure, I need information from different sources for my report, and they need to be referenced and research based, my teacher said."

"No problem. I'll show you how to navigate MedlinePlus and then I'll be back in a few minutes to see if you're ready for the books and journals. How does that sound?" asked Jenny.

"Great—thanks for your help!" the boy responded.

TABLE 10.4
Teen Health Resources

Girl's Health
http://www.girlshealth.gov/index.html
  This website developed by the Office on Women's Health in the Department of
Health & Human Services provides girls ages ten through sixteen information that
promotes healthy behaviors with tips on health and relationships.

Planned Parenthood Info for Teens
http://www.plannedparenthood.org/info-for-teens/
  Information from Planned Parenthood on the questions teens ask about sex,
relationships, and their bodies. Includes information and tools for parents and
educators.

Teen Health from MedlinePlus
http://www.nlm.nih.gov/medlineplus/teenhealth.html
  From the National Library of Medicine, this MedlinePlus teen health page includes
information of interest to teens including body image, alcohol and drug use, nutrition,
sexuality, and more.

Teen Health FX
http://www.teenhealthfx.com/
  An award-winning teen health website on topics about health, relationships, physical
development, and sexuality. Funded by the Atlantic Health System's Morristown
Medical Center.

TeensHealth
http://teenshealth.org/teen/
  This is the teen health section of the KidsHealth website from Nemours Foundation.
A team of pediatricians and medical experts review the content regularly to ensure
accuracy.

Meeting the Information Needs of the LGBT Community

In the United States, this is a time of progressively rapid enlightenment with
changes in attitudes and legislation regarding equality for the LGBT community. Marriage equality is now law in many states, and gay people may
serve openly and honorably in the military. But even so, health disparities
still plague this community. Discrimination, stigma, fear, and a lack of knowledge on the part of healthcare providers continue to be a challenge for LGBT
people when it comes to their health.

  Consumer health libraries have a role to play in the provision of health
information that can improve, and in some cases, literally save the lives of
LGBT individuals. Healthcare providers and librarians alike are front and
center when it comes to helping to answer questions not only for LGBT
people, but their family members and allies. Research shows that LGBT per-

sons share a disproportionate amount of health issues due to stigmatization and discrimination. This includes the fact that a large number of healthcare providers lack the knowledge and cultural competence needed to care for these individuals and their particular health concerns (McKay, 2011). Lack of providers' knowledge and cultural competence adds to the reluctance of LGBT persons to seek preventive services. In turn, this leads to increased rates of a range of mental health issues, among them depression, anxiety, and suicide, as well as a delay in routine medical care related to physical health. These health disparities are particularly prevalent in rural areas of the country where many LGBT people continue to feel isolated. In rural areas, it can be difficult to locate LGBT-friendly providers as well as helpful community resources. Yet, there is good news for this frequently under-served community. Governmental and healthcare institutions recognize the issue and are working to address it. In 2011, the Institute of Medicine released a report titled *The Health of Lesbian, Gay, Bisexual and Transgender People: Building a Foundation for Better Understanding*, and the Joint Commission, the powerful and influential not-for-profit organization that accredits and certifies hospitals across the nation, published *Advancing Effective Communication, Cultural Competence, and Patient and Family-Centered Care for the Lesbian, Gay, Bisexual, and Transgendered (LGBT) Community* to assist the healthcare community in improving the quality of care and services for this group of consumers. Both publications provide guidelines, resource guides, and checklists with valuable information to increase communication and cultural competence and the overall treatment and care of LGBT persons.

Consumer health libraries can effectively work with this community by training staff to be culturally competent and knowledgeable about resources available. Creating an atmosphere that projects inclusiveness incorporates the physical environment as well as library staff who are able to make LGBT consumers comfortable through the language they use and attitudes that de-note respect. If the library doesn't project a welcoming environment, even a high-quality collection will fail to compensate.

Consumer health libraries may utilize signs and symbols signifying they are LGBT-friendly and welcoming. These can be subtle, but they speak volumes about the library's non-verbal support:

- Post a rainbow, pink triangle, or LGBT organization logo symbol on a door or window.
- Display a non-discrimination statement in a visible place in the library.
- Hang posters or pictures depicting a variety of diverse people and fami-lies or promoting organizations that provide support and information

(i.e., local PFLAG [Parents, Family and Friends of Lesbians, Gays including bisexual and transgender persons]).

- Add LGBT-specific health brochures and publications to handout materials (multilingual when possible).
- Include links to LGBT health organizations and resources in the library website's health links.
- Provide a gender-neutral restroom. This is very much appreciated by transgender people and others who don't conform to gender stereotypes.

Of course, all the symbols and efforts to create an inclusive atmosphere will be for naught if staff does not project a corresponding welcome and sensitivity. Staff must feel confident with their ability to interact with any and all customers. Providing ongoing training in this particular aspect of cultural competency is important to give staff the skills and comfort level needed to provide meaningful health information. Some ways to support cultural competence and sensitivity training include the following:

- Enlist the assistance of an openly gay, lesbian, bisexual, or transgender employee. They can provide valuable knowledge and perspectives about serving this community.
- Provide training about homophobia and LGBT health concerns. Every employee should be aware of online and local resources.
- Teach staff appropriate language to use when addressing LGBT people.
- If there is a local PFLAG or other LGBT support group, find out how the library can be included in their list of resources. Go speak at one of their meetings about the valuable information that can be found at the consumer health library.
- Post LGBT support group information in highly visible areas of the consumer health library. For LGBT people newly located to an area, attending a local support group is a great way to meet likeminded people in their new community.
- If high schools in the area sponsor Gay-Straight Alliances, provide a list of LGBT resources available at the consumer health library to these groups.

Equality for the LGBT community is moving steadily forward, but for gay and lesbian Americans there remains stigma associated with sexual orientation in many areas of the country and that includes healthcare. Through developing culturally competent staff, promoting services provided by the consumer health library, as well as creating an environment that is welcoming and inviting, consumer health librarians are able to provide essential information vital to the health and well-being of this community.

Strategies for a successful interaction include the following:

- Thank patrons for noticing the library's LGBT window stickers.
- If there is an openly gay staff member, this individual may be a useful resource for an LGBT patron's question.
- Ask if an LGBT patron is interested in contact information about the nearest local PFLAG support group.
- Introduce the patron to the Gay and Lesbian Medical Association—Health Professionals Advancing LGBT Equality and their "Find a Provider" online provider directory.
- Introduce the patron to other LGBT publications and brochures in the library.

TABLE 10.5
Snapshot of Strategies in Action: Successful Interaction for LGBT Health Information

It had been a busy afternoon and Mary was finally getting a break in the action to fill some book holds at the reference desk one afternoon when a young man approached her. Mary looked up from the computer screen, "Hello, what can I help you with today?" Mary asked with a smile.

"Hi," the young man replied in a friendly voice. "I'm not sure you can help me, but I noticed the stickers in your window and thought, 'Why not ask?' I just moved from out-of-state to Jonesville to work for Hashtag.com, you know the business that just opened recently? Anyway, I have a question related to those stickers. I'd like to find a doctor here locally, but it's important to me that I find someone who has a gay-friendly practice and will be comfortable treating me. In the area I used to live in, it was easy to locate doctors who treated gay people. In fact, most of their patients were gay. But here, I don't really know anyone to ask. Is there anything in this library that might help me to find a new doctor here?"

"Well," said Mary with a pleased tone, "I'm really glad you noticed those stickers—and, that they brought you in. We have a staff member who is very knowledgeable about the gay community here locally. Do you mind if I ask her to assist?"

"No, not at all—that would be great!" said the young man.

Mary asked Janice, an out LGBT staff member, if she had time to assist. "Hi, I think I might know of some resources that will be really useful," said Janice. "Let's start with the healthcare question, shall we? There's a website called GLMA. Are you familiar with it?"

"No, I don't think I've heard of that before. What is it?" he asked.

Janice led the young man towards the public Internet stations and explained that it is the Gay and Lesbian Medical Association, which has a great tool called a "provider directory" to locate gay-friendly healthcare providers in the local area. "I'll show you how to use the directory. What other questions do you have about your new community?" she asked. "I know there are some local support and social groups in the area, PFLAG being one, and we have some of their brochures. I'd be happy to show you those when you're ready. I'll check back in a few minutes to see how you're doing."

TABLE 10.6
LGBT Resources

AIDS Info
http://aidsinfo.nih.gov/
Offers information and fact sheets on HIV/AIDS treatment, prevention, and research.

Centers for Disease Control and Prevention LGBT Health
http://www.cdc.gov/lgbthealth/
Centers for Disease Control and Prevention LGBT content-rich website section.

Gay and Lesbian Medical Association (GLMA)
Health Professionals Advancing LGBT Equality
http://glma.org/
GLMA's mission is to ensure equality in healthcare for lesbian, gay, bisexual, and transgender (LGBT) individuals and healthcare providers. Includes an LGBT-friendly provider directory.

MedlinePlus
http://www.nlm.nih.gov/medlineplus/gaylesbianbisexualandtransgenderhealth.html
MedlinePlus from the National Library of Medicine information on LGBT health.

National LGBT Health Education Center of the Fenway Institute
http://www.lgbthealtheducation.org/
The National LGBT Health Education Center provides programs for healthcare organizations to reduce health disparities among LGBT individuals.

Out for Health
http://www.outforhealth.org/healthy-people-2020.html
Planned Parenthood's LGBT Health and Wellness Project provides outreach, education, and information to the LGBT community.

PFLAG National
http://community.pflag.org/
PFLAG (Parents, Families and Friends of Lesbians and Gays) is a national support, education, and advocacy nonprofit organization formed to support the LGBT community.

Rainbow Access Initiative
http://rainbowaccess.org/
The Rainbow Access Initiative is an all-volunteer organization to help educate healthcare professionals and ensure the LGBT community receives culturally competent care.

Meeting the Needs of Special Groups and Underserved Populations

Providing quality health information for those with limited English proficiency (LEP) and low health literacy may also pose special challenges for the consumer health librarian. While outreach to underserved populations is a mission of many consumer health libraries, it can be a daunting task. The lack of accessible and understandable health information for the diverse populations in the United States is a barrier to health literacy and affects the health of millions of people. This issue of healthcare inequity affects not only LEP and low literate people, but also people with disabilities and their caregivers. The Agency for Healthcare Research and Quality states that health disparities disproportionately affect minority groups, people with disabilities, those with limited income and education, and rural residents (Geiger et al., 2010). Healthcare inequity also affects the large population of Baby Boomers, also known as the graying of America. As of 2010, 40.4 million people in the United States were sixty-five years of age or older. The number is expected to increase to 72.1 million by 2030 (Gerontology Society of America, 2012). The problem is not just limited to the individuals in these populations seeking information to help them make sense of their health conditions, but also to healthcare providers, whose inadequate communication with these individuals leads to poor health outcomes, hospital readmissions, or adverse events.

Studies show that people with LEP and low health literacy have less knowledge about their conditions, don't take advantage of preventive care, are at risk for prescription medication errors, and are more frequently hospitalized. In addition to the human toll, these factors have a huge financial impact on healthcare organizations and our nation as a whole.

According to the Institute of Medicine, nearly *half* the adult population in the United States has difficulty accessing health information and services. The Medical Library Association's Health Literacy Task Force created a definition for "health information literacy" as "the set of abilities needed to recognize a health information need, identify likely information sources and use them to retrieve relevant information, assess the quality of the information and its applicability to a specific situation, and analyze, understand, and use the information to make good health decisions" (Shipman et al., 2009, p. 294). The challenge for consumer health librarians is twofold. First is training healthcare providers and allied health personnel about the harmful consequences of low health literacy, the importance of clear communication which includes providing understandable health information, and the valuable services librarians deliver to support this effort. Second is offering adequate resources and education directly to this vulnerable population. Doing so may improve their health literacy and help them better manage their health. This is especially important as more responsibility for health decisions and cost is shifted to individuals. Recent data showed 55 percent of healthcare expenses in the United States are paid for by individuals themselves, and 35 percent of the population either did not have health insurance or had inadequate coverage (Garcia-Retamero and Galesic, 2009). Many of the uninsured and underinsured people in the United States are the working poor, LEP, or low literate.

Fortunately, there are tools, resources, and strategies to assist in both the effort to raise awareness about health literacy barriers among healthcare professionals and provide appropriate health information within the library to these special populations. These include the use of culturally appropriate audio and video recordings, picture books, easy-to-read written materials, and a variety of multilingual Internet websites and online low literate health information. Other means include building a collection of materials around the prevalent minority population(s) reflected in the community. Forging connections and building relationships with members from those communities opens the door to asking them for insight into the needs and cultural norms of the group. Health departments, churches, schools, and senior centers are excellent places to learn about the diverse groups and predominant cultures within the community. These locations are also excellent places to provide information about the valuable services and materials for underserved populations available through the consumer health library. Inviting local support and English-as-a-second-language groups to meet in your facility offers a wonderful opportunity to introduce consumer health materials and resources. Individuals often feel more comfortable in a group of people who share common concerns and issues, and may be more likely to ask questions and seek assistance from staff in a support group setting.

As technology advances and healthcare organizations incorporate the use of electronic medical records, electronic health records, and the subsequent utilization of patient portals, consumer health librarians have a perfect opportunity to use their expert searching and teaching skills to assist many LEP, elderly, and low-literate individuals to register and navigate the patient portal environment.

As always, the consumer health library environment must convey a sense of welcoming to any and all who enter the door. It's important for helpful and knowledgeable staff to convey compassion and patience, essential elements when working with LEP, elderly, and low-literate people. Identifying staff members who are fluent in a particular language through pins or buttons (e.g., "Se habla Español") can be an effective means of connection for LEP patrons who may already feel uncertain and insecure about how or who to approach in the library.

As the information environment becomes continually more complex, reaching these often difficult-to-access groups is challenging yet crucial and can be a very rewarding and satisfying aspect of being a consumer health librarian. When budgets and resources are squeezed, programs and partnerships that open and expand access to collections, such as library consortiums consisting of public, private, and special libraries, greatly enhance the ability of patrons to locate health information and increase the visibility of the consumer health library in the larger community. By joining together, library partnerships are stronger and better able to serve those who need access to information the most.

Technology continues to evolve and improve access to information, helping to reduce health disparities for LEP and low health literacy individuals.

While resources may not be evolving at the rate of technology, they, too, are improving the ability to find health information in a variety languages and formats. Such advances assist consumer health librarians in delivering health information that is culturally and linguistically relevant, easy-to-read for those with limited reading skills, and available in multiple formats to benefit the diverse populations we serve.

Strategies for a successful interaction include the following:

- Take the patron(s) to a quiet area away from other library patrons and speak quietly to ensure their privacy.
- Listen carefully and patiently to their concerns.
- Repeat back to the patron in simple terms your understanding of their question.
- Clarify anything you don't understand.

TABLE 10.7
Snapshot of Strategies in Action: Meeting the
Needs of Special Groups and Underserved Populations

Ann was working one morning when she heard some familiar voices, but they sounded upset. Looking up, she saw Camille and Sonya, but they were not looking or sounding happy. Ann quietly and calmly greeted the two women who were well known to all the staff. "Hello, you seem upset, how can I help you today?" asked Ann.

"Oh, Ann, we just learned that if we don't answer a questionnaire on the computer, our health insurance will cost us a lot more this season. We can't afford that, but we don't have a computer and we don't know how to use one! They said someone at work could help us, but we don't want anyone there knowing anything about our private health information," Camille replied anxiously.

Ann nodded in understanding and moved around the desk to face them. "Let's go over to this table where we can talk privately." Once they were seated, Ann asked, "How can we help you?"

"Can you get us signed up on the computer and help us fill out the questionnaire they're talking about?" the women asked. "We have the instructions here. It says we need a password or something—how do we do that?"

"You said you have the instructions with you. May I look at them?" asked Ann. "Hmm, I see, it says you will both need to register on the computer using your name and a password you make up that you'll be able to remember. Once you do that you can sign onto the website where the questionnaire is located. I believe we have a computer back in the corner that is available. This will take some time, but I think we can walk you through registering on the website and answering the questionnaire. First, let me see if I can find someone to cover the desk. Does that sound all right to you?"

"Yes, thank you so much, Ann! We weren't sure what we were going to do if we couldn't get help here," replied Sonya.

TABLE 10.8
Multi-Lingual Resources for LEP Patrons

Health Information in Your Language
http://health.qld.gov.au/multicultural/public/language.asp#links
   Sponsored by Queensland Health in Australia. Provides multilingual health information by topic and language, as well as links to translated health information from other websites.

Life with Cancer
http://www.lifewithcancer.org/managing_symptoms.php
   Life with Cancer is sponsored by northern Virginia's Inova Health System. These fact sheets offer information in twelve languages about managing common symptoms and side effects of cancer treatment.

Multicultural Health Communications Services
http://www.mhcs.health.nsw.gov.au/
   This is a website developed by the Multicultural Health Communication Service of New South Wales, Australia, for people working with culturally and linguistically diverse populations. They offer health information in multiple languages and formats.

NNLM Consumer Health Information in Many Languages Resources
http://nnlm.gov/outreach/consumer/multi.html
   The National Network of Libraries of Medicine offers this extensive list of links to resources in a variety of languages.

(See more resources referenced in Chapter 11.)

TABLE 10.9
General Resources for Plain Language Health Information

American Academy of Family Physicians
http://familydoctor.org/
Easy-to-read information on diseases and conditions, prevention, wellness, and specific age groups. Spanish language available.

Consumer and Patient Health Information Section of the Medical Library Association
http://caphis.mlanet.org/consumer/
Provides a top one hundred list of recommended websites for consumer health information, including general health as well as websites geared towards specific groups.

Healthfinder.gov
http://healthfinder.gov/
Healthfinder is a gateway consumer health information from the U.S. Department of Health and Human Services. Healthfinder's "Health A–Z" provides information on over 1,600 different health topics. Spanish language available.

Health Radio
http://www.healthradio.net/
Health Radio is an online talk radio portal for health, wellness, medical news, and information. The website provides links to audio podcasts and video interviews with physicians, research scientists, authors, and other experts in various fields of medicine and health. Health Radio has affiliations with the American Academy of Pediatrics and other medical organizations. They are funded through promotion and advertising sales.

Mayo Clinic
http://www.mayoclinic.com/
From the Mayo Clinic, find comprehensive consumer health information on hundreds of conditions, drugs, tests and procedures, and even healthy recipes.

MedlinePlus
http://www.nlm.nih.gov/medlineplus/
MedlinePlus from the National Library of Medicine is a one-stop shopping website for up-to-date, reliable health information in multiple languages and formats, including easy-to-read. MedlinePlus provides information on health topics, medicine, and health directories.

National Institutes of Diabetes and Digestive and Kidney Diseases
http://www2.niddk.nih.gov/HealthEducation/HealthEzToRead.htm
From the National Institutes of Health. Easy-to-read publications on diabetes and digestive and kidney diseases. Many of the publications are available in Spanish.

TABLE 10.10
Resources for Learning More about Underserved Populations

Centers for Disease Control and Prevention. "Health Literacy: Accurate, Accessible, and Actionable Health Information for All." http://www.cdc.gov/healthliteracy/.

Culture Clues. *Patient and Family Education Services. A Department of University of Washington Medical Center.* http://depts.washington.edu/pfes/CultureClues.htm.

DeWalt, DA, et al. *Health Literacy Universal Precautions Toolkit.* (Prepared by North Carolina Network Consortium, The Cecil G. Sheps Center for Health Services Research, University of North Carolina at Chapel Hill, under Contract No. HHSA290200710014.) AHRQ Publication No. 10-0046-EF). Rockville, MD: Agency for Healthcare Research and Quality, 2010.

Gay & Lesbian Medical Association. *Guidelines for Care of Lesbian, Gay, Bisexual, and Transgender Patients.* San Francisco: GLMA, 2006. http://www.glma.org/index .cfm?fuseaction=Page.viewPage&pageId=622&parentID=534&nodeID=1.

Ham, K. *Finding Health and Wellness @ the Library: A Consumer Health Toolkit for Library Staff.* 2nd edition. A project of California State Library and NN/LM, 2013. http://www.library.ca.gov/lds/docs/healthtoolkit.pdf.

The Joint Commission. *Advancing Effective Communication, Cultural Competence, and Patient-and Family-Centered Care for the Lesbian, Gay, Bisexual, and Transgender (LGBT) Community: A Field Guide.* Oak Brook, IL: The Joint Commission, October 2011. LGBTFieldGuide.pdf.

Kars, M, Baker, LM, and Wilson, FL, eds. *Medical Library Association Guide to Health Literacy.* New York: Neal-Schuman, 2008.

Medical Library Association Health Information Literacy (Health Information Literacy Curriculum). http://mlanet.org/resources/healthlit/.

Spatz, M. *Answering Consumer Health Questions: The Medical Library Association Guide for Reference Librarians.* New York: Neal Schuman, 2008.

U.S. Department of Health and Human Services, Office of Disease Prevention and Health Promotion. *National Action Plan to Improve Health Literacy.* Washington, DC: U.S. Department of Health and Human Services, 2010.

Wilson-Stronks, A, et al. *One Size Does Not Fit All: Meeting the Health Care Needs of Diverse Populations.* Oakbrook Terrace, IL: The Joint Commission, 2008.

References

Alpi, K, and Bibel, B. 2004. "Meeting the Health Information Needs of Diverse Populations." *Library Trends*, Fall:270–82.

Borzekowski, D, et al. 2012. "Ten Years of TeenHealthFX.com: A Case Study of an Adolescent Health Web Site." *Pediatric Clinics of North America*, 59:717–27.

Garcia-Retamero, R, and Galesic, M. 2009. "Communicating Treatment Risk Reduction to People with Low Numeracy Skills: A Cross-Cultural Comparison." *American Journal of Public Health*, 99(12):2196–202.

Geiger, B, et al. 2010. "Responding to Health Information and Training Needs of Individuals with Disabilities." *Journal of Consumer Health on the Internet*, 40(1):22–32.

Gerontology Society of America. 2012. *Communicating with Older Adults: An Evidence-Based Review of What Really Works.* Washington, DC: The Gerontology Society of America.

Ghaddar, S, et al. 2011. "Adolescent Health Literacy: The Importance of Credible Sources for Online Health Information." *Journal of School Health*, 82(1):28–36.

Gibbons, M. 2011. "Use of Health Information Technology among Racial and Ethnic Underserved Communities." *Perspectives in Health Information Management*, Winter:1–13.

McKay, B. 2011. "Lesbian, Gay, Bisexual, and Transgender Health Issues, Disparities, and Information Resources." *Medical References Services Quarterly*, 30(4):394.

Paek, HJ, and Hove, T. 2012. "Social Cognitive Factors and Perceived Social Influences That Improve Adolescent eHealth Literacy." *Health Communications*, 27:727–37.

Parker, R. 2000. "Health Literacy: A Challenge for American Patients and Their Health Care Providers." *Health Promotion International*, 15(4):277–83.

Parker, R, and Kreps, G. 2005. "Library Outreach: Overcoming Health Literacy Challenges." *Journal of the Medical Library Association*, 93(4):S81–S85.

Purnell, L, and Paulanka, B. 2008. *Transcultural Health Care: A Culturally Competent Approach.* Philadelphia, PA: F.A. Davis Co.

Sentell, T, and Braun, K. 2012. "Low Health Literacy, Limited English Proficiency, and Health Status in Asians, Latinos, and Other Racial/Ethnic Groups in California." *Journal of Health Communication*, 17(Suppl 3):82–99.

Shipman, J, et al. 2009. "The Health Information Literacy Research Project." *Journal of the Medical Library Association*, 97(4):293–301.

Smart, K, et al. 2012. "Speaking Up: Teens Voice Their Health Information Needs." *The Journal of School Nursing*, 28(5):379–88.

Spatz, M. 2008. *Answering Consumer Health Questions: The Medical Library Association Guide for Reference Librarians.* New York: Neal-Schuman.

U.S. Department of Health and Human Services, Office of Disease Prevention and Health Promotion. 2010. *National Action Plan to Improve Health Literacy.* Washington, DC: U.S. Department of Health and Human Services.

11

Cultural Sensitivity and Health Information Resources and Services

Donna J. McCloskey

IN SOCIETIES WHERE PEOPLE ARE INCREASINGLY mobile throughout the world, the possibility exists that a medical librarian will encounter a patron who has emigrated from a different country and culture than the librarian's own. The challenge for information professionals is to provide authoritative and reliable health information to these patrons in a caring and sensitive manner. Even more important than information "are awareness, respect, and acceptance of the client's cultural beliefs and practices as equally valid as your own" (U.S. Department of Agriculture, 1986).

The United States has always been a melting pot, and community demographics has always played an important role in how librarians respond to their patrons' needs for health information. According to *The World Factbook*, the population of the United States is "white 79.96%, black 12.85%, Asian 4.43%, Amerindian and Alaska native 0.97%, native Hawaiian and other Pacific Islanders 0.18%" (Central Intelligence Agency, 2013). It should be noted that the Hispanic population is not listed separately because the U.S. Census Bureau considers Hispanic to encompass persons of different origins, including Mexican and Spanish, who may be any race or ethnic group. According to the U.S. Census Bureau, the Hispanic population is projected to more than double by 2060 with nearly one in three U.S. residents of Hispanic origin, up from one in six in 2012. Overall, minorities, which are now 37 percent of the population, are projected to rise to 57 percent by 2060 (U.S. Census Bureau, 2012). In addition, the U.S. Census Bureau's 2010 American Community Survey identified and recorded seventy nationalities within the total population with German, Irish, English, and Italian topping the list followed by French,

Scottish, Dutch, and Norwegian (U.S. Census Bureau, 2010). *The World Fact-book* estimates that the net migration rate (number of persons entering the country per year per one thousand persons) will be 3.64 for 2013, which ranks the United States as twenty-eighth in the world (Central Intelligence Agency, 2013). With statistics such as these, it is imperative that medical librarians create an environment where persons from divergent cultures can obtain authoritative consumer and patient health information without bias.

A culturally sensitive person is one who possesses basic knowledge of and constructive attitudes towards the health and health traditions observed among diverse cultural groups found in his or her community (Spector, 2013, p. 11). What are the standards surrounding this concept and how do librarians ensure that they are indeed culturally sensitive?

The National Standards for Culturally and Linguistically Appropriate Services (CLAS) in Health and Health Care were initially adopted by the U.S. Department of Health and Human Services, Office of Minority Health, in 2001. In 2010, the Office of Minority Health launched the National CLAS Standards Enhancement Initiative with the goal of expanding the scope of the standards and improving clarity to ensure understanding and implementation. The new, enhanced national standards were revealed in April 2013. The standards are primarily directed at healthcare organizations but are certainly appropriate for librarians to integrate into their services as well. The Principal Standard and the three standards under Governance, Leadership, and Workforce are particularly important to consider:

Principal Standard:

1. Provide effective, equitable, understandable, and respectful quality of care and services that are responsive to diverse cultural health beliefs and practices, preferred languages, health literacy, and other communication needs.

Governance, Leadership, and Workforce:

2. Advance and sustain organizational governance and leadership that promotes CLAS and health equity through policy, practices, and allocated resources.
3. Recruit, promote, and support a culturally and linguistically diverse governance, leadership, and workforce that are responsive to the population in the service area.
4. Educate and train governance, leadership, and workforce in culturally and linguistically appropriate policies and practices on an ongoing basis

(U.S. Department of Health and Human Services, Office of Minority Health, Think Cultural Health, 2013).

Additionally, the CLAS Standards recommend maintaining accurate and reliable demographic data and conducting regular assessments of community health assets and needs.

It is the responsibility of all medical librarians and managers of library staff to ensure that both they and their staff make a commitment to cultural sensitivity. The understanding of cultural values and beliefs will result in more positive interaction with patrons. Some basic components of this commitment include asking patrons how they would like to be addressed, why they have come to the library, and what the goal is for their visit. Demonstrating understanding and respect can go a long way in building trusting interactions with patrons (University of Washington Medical Center, Patient and Family Education Services, 2011). Asking for help in understanding another's culture demonstrates sincere openness, a desire to learn, and shows respect for the patron's culture (Diller, 2004, p. 155).

Medical librarians must possess an attitude that reflects an awareness of the impact of cultural factors, the need to avoid stereotyping, the recognition of one's own personal biases, a respect and tolerance for cultural differences, and the ethical obligation to challenge discrimination (Like, Steiner, and Rubel, 1996, p. 292).

The following websites are helpful resources for medical library staff in understanding and learning about cultural sensitivity.

While the reference interview is nothing new to librarians, conducting an interview with a person from another culture requires special strategies. Techniques and models used by medical professionals can be adapted for use by the medical librarians.

One such model is referred to by the mnemonic LEARN. This guideline includes:

Listening to the patron's perspective
Explaining one's own perspective
Acknowledging differences and similarities between the two perspectives
Recommending options, and
Negotiating differences (Juckett, 2013, p. 52).

The ETHNIC mnemonic is another tool that can be used to demonstrate cultural sensitivity and aid in the reference interview process. This process begins by asking three questions:

TABLE 11.1
Websites for Understanding and Learning about Cultural Sensitivity

CulturedMed http://culturedmed.binghamton.edu	The underlying mission of the CulturedMed project, which focuses on provision of culturally competent healthcare to refugees and immigrants worldwide, is: "our ability to recognize the cultural assumptions of others is contingent upon our awareness of our own assumptions." The website includes a wide range of bibliographies on diverse topics; currently, there are ten thousand citations.
DiversityRx http://diversityrx.org	DiversityRx exists to "improve the accessibility and quality of health care for minority, immigrant, and indigenous families." The organization's website is an excellent place to keep abreast of information on best practices. Key topics include culturally competent care and language access; an organization directory is a wealth of resources. In addition, one may join the Culturally and Linguistically Appropriate Services–talk email discussion group from this website. This listserv addresses many aspects of cross-cultural health and can be a resource for locating information.
EthnoMed http://ethnomed.org	EthnoMed covers medical and cultural information on fifteen immigrant and refugee groups plus a collection of resources related to cross-cultural health.
Office of Minority Health http://minorityhealth.hhs.gov	This government agency is dedicated to eliminating health disparities and improving health. The website provides statistics and information on minority populations in the United States. Maps display states where the largest populations of various minorities reside. A searchable Knowledge Center Library is also available. Cultural Competence is a key searchable subject term in the library's database.
Outreach Activities and Resources http://sis.nlm.nih.gov/outreach.html	The Specialized Information Services branch of the National Library of Medicine has compiled Multi-Cultural Resources for Health Information from this fundamental website. Resources range from cultural competency to health resources in other languages to refugee health portals.

How do you Explain your illness?
What Treatment have you tried?
Have you sought any advice from folk Healers?

These questions are followed by:

Negotiating options,
Agreeing upon Intervention, and
Collaboration with family and possibly healers (Medical University of South Carolina, College of Medicine, 2013).

For many cultures, it is particularly important to include the family as health-care decisions may be made by the family as a whole or the husband of female patients.

A simple model that can be used in the course of the reference interview is called the 4 Cs of Culture. It consists of the following questions:

What do you call your problem?
What do you think caused it?
What have you done to cope with it?
What concerns you about it?
What concerns do you have about treatment? (Galanti, 2008, p. 250).

The goals of an initial meeting with a patron should include establishing a good rapport, understanding the patron's problem and expectations, communicating clearly what can be offered, and providing the patron with the experience of being heard. These are not unlike the goals of a reference interview where no cultural differences exist. However, a more extensive questioning may be necessary to adequately address the concerns of the patrons. The medical librarian may wish to ask questions about the family structure, language spoken at home, economic situation, education level, amount of acculturation, traditions practiced at home, religion, and community patterns (Diller, 2004, p. 153).

It is important for the medical librarian to realize that non-verbal communication may mean different things in different cultures. The Chinese prefer a respectful seating distance and may prefer to sit side by side (Lipson and Dibble, 2008, p. 100). Allow the patron to choose seating for comfortable personal space and eye contact. Hmong consider finger pointing at an adult as rude (Lipson and Dibble, 2008, p. 253). Avoid body language that may be misunderstood or offensive. Silence for Arabs may indicate respect but not necessarily agreement (Lipson and Dibble, 2008, p. 45). Do not assume that silence means that the patron is not listening; check for understanding (Spector, 2013, p. 326).

In order for medical library staff to follow through with providing culturally sensitive health information, easy access to resources with cultural information must be available for staff to acquire a basic knowledge of cultural values and health beliefs. There are several excellent print resources for this purpose.

Mosby's *Pocket Guide to Cultural Health Assessment* (D'Avanzo, 2008) addresses a growing world where the library patron population is more diverse and requires a greater understanding and tolerance of different ways of life. Just as people may dress and speak differently, their approach to health information may be different as well. Cultural competence for librarians encompasses basic cultural, epidemiological, environmental, and geographical information.

Being culturally competent in the cultures that a librarian may routinely encounter is important. Aside from print resources such as the *Pocket Guide to Cultural Health Assessment*, a recommendation is made to achieve greater understanding of cultural groups in the local region through media and research studies. Going to markets in ethnic neighborhoods, attending religious ceremonies, and attending life celebrations such as weddings and graduations are wonderful ways to get a sense of community and cultural difference (D'Avanzo, 2008, p. xviii).

Mosby's *Pocket Guide to Cultural Health Assessment*'s contributing authors represent countries worldwide. The number of countries covered in the book numbers nearly two hundred. Each country's location; major languages, ethnic groups, and religions; healthcare beliefs; predominant sick-care practices; ethnic-/race-specific or endemic diseases; health-team relationships; families' role in hospital care; dominance patterns; eye-contact practices; touch practices; perceptions of time; pain reactions; birth and death rites; food practices and intolerances; infant-feeding practices; child-rearing practices; and national childhood immunizations are all addressed.

Culture & Clinical Care (Lipson and Dibble, 2008) covers the thirty-five most populous countries represented in the United States, according to the U.S. Census. Of particular importance is the time of arrival in the United States of emigrates. This impacts acculturation, communication, and health beliefs and practices. The following are taken into consideration for each country: cultural/ethnic identity, spiritual/religious orientation, oral and non-verbal communication preferences, activities of daily living, food practices, symptom management, birth ritual, developmental and sexual issues, family relationships, illness beliefs, health issues, and death rituals. Each country's section is also followed up with selected references.

Cultural Diversity in Health and Illness (Spector, 2013) focuses on the major ethnic populations of the United States in expanded chapters within the book. Emphasis is placed on American Indian, Alaska Native, Asian, black, Hispanic, and white populations. The appendixes of this book include a "Quick Guide for Cultural Care" and a set of questions titled the "Heritage Assessment Tool." This tool can also be helpful in assessing and understanding one's own health beliefs and practices.

In addition to these selected print resources, there are a number of electronic resources to guide librarians in gaining knowledge of ethnic groups and accessing health information in various languages.

To demonstrate the healthcare distinctions between ethnic populations, consider how Afghan, African American, Chinese, German, Hmong, Mexican, and Vietnamese cultures differ as they relate to perception of pain and causes of physical illness. See table 11.2.

TABLE 11.2
Cultural Differences in Perception and Causes of Pain

Culture	Perception of Pain	Causes of Physical Illness
Afghans	Elderly may see pain as God's punishment or as an expected part of life; non-pharmacological method for reducing pain is to listen to the Koran	Illness can have natural causes such as germs or seasonal changes
African Americans	Expression of pain generally open; all forms of pain management acceptable	View illness as a state of disharmony; may view as God's punishment for improper behavior
Chinese	Patient may not complain of pain; may use acupuncture to treat pain	Imbalance of yin and yang
Germans	Tend to be stoic and may not report pain or ask for pain medication	Most believe that poor nutrition, stress, or inadequate rest cause illness
Hmong	Do not use pain scales well; readily accept analgesic medications	Believe that illness can have natural or supernatural etiologies
Mexicans	May want pain relief as quickly as possible	May view physical illness as an act of God
Vietnamese	Maintain self-control and do not complain	Belief in spiritual causes is common; will not reveal such beliefs to Western healthcare professionals

Source: Lipson and Dibble, 2008.

TABLE 11.3
Websites for Health Information in Other Languages

Consumer Health Information in Many Languages Resources http://www.nnlm.gov/outreach/consumer/multi.html	From a collaboration of the National Network of Libraries of Medicine Consumer Outreach Librarians, links to resources in multiple languages as well as for specific languages are compiled.
DeafMD.org http://www.deafmd.org	Health Information in American Sign Language is accessible from alphabetical listings of diseases and diagnostic tests. There is also an option to search for a deaf-friendly physician.
EthnoMed http://www.ethnomed.org/patient-education	This website includes sections searchable by health topic and language and an annotated listing of related websites.
Health Information Translations http://healthinfotranslations.org	Easy-to-read and culturally appropriate education resources are provided and searchable by keywords, health topic, or language. Some topics are available with audio and video translations.
Healthy Roads Media http://www.healthyroadsmedia.org	Health information is searchable by topic or language in a variety of formats, including a mobile application.
MedlinePlus Health Information in Multiple Languages http://www.nlm.nih.gov/medlineplus/languages/languages.html	Health information in fifty languages is available and searchable by language or health topic.
Office of Minority Health, Knowledge Center Library http://minorityhealth.hhs.gov Click on "Search Library Catalog" on the left-hand column.	The Knowledge Center Library online catalog includes consumer health materials in over thirty-five different languages. Select "Advanced Search" and enter the desired language to find these materials.
Refugee Health Information Network http://rhin.org	An advanced search capability that includes language, format, and category makes this website particularly valuable for locating multilingual health information for refugees.
Selected Patient Information Resources in Asian Languages (SPIRAL) http://spiral.tufts.edu/index.php	Patient information resources in Asian languages are provided with the source for each health topic documented.

Since its opening nearly twenty years ago, the health library at Novant Health Matthews Medical Center in Matthews, North Carolina, has served patients within the hospital as well as the community in which it resides and beyond (Byrd and Caddell, 2013). Matthews is a town of just under thirty thousand people and a suburb of Charlotte. Both communities have a predominantly white population with African American and Hispanic as the next largest demographic groups (U.S. Census Bureau, 2013).

The library staff is fortunate to receive diversity training, a requirement of all Novant Health employees in support of one of the corporation's values: diversity. The healthcare organization recognizes that every person is different and shaped by unique life experiences. As part of this training, staff completes a diversity self-assessment.

The medical librarian and staff at Novant Health Matthews Medical Center develop trust with patrons seeking health information by first observing and listening to people, being sensitive to where they are in their health journey continuum, and then offering assistance as they know people are ready to learn more about their health condition. Sometimes this means saying, "Okay, I'll check on you later."

When a staff member has established a relationship with a specific patron, every effort is made for that staff member to handle the patron's questions going forward, even though another staff member may be equally capable. Another key component to building trust is to follow up with patrons, making the personal connection even stronger.

For inpatients, the medical librarian has a method for approaching them and their families. When rounding on inpatients in the hospital, the librarian begins by sitting down in the room if possible, introducing herself to the patient and his or her family, and simply saying that she is there to check on them and see if they need anything. She explains the services that the library can offer from evidence-based health information to support groups to physician referrals. Even though the librarian may know the patient's diagnosis, she lets the patient say and approach the topic first.

The health library at Novant Health Matthews Medical Center also uses trained volunteers to work with patients. At times, these volunteers are matched with patients due to a specialized skill that the volunteer may have. One volunteer may be paired with a patient who is particularly anxious because she is good at alleviating fears, while another works with a patient with a critical condition because that volunteer has personal experience with a critical health situation of his own and can relate.

Building relationships within the community is another key aspect of the library's services. The healthcare organization has a Community Care Cruiser that provides primary care, immunizations, and routine check-ups to uninsured and underinsured youth in the community by way of a traveling

Bright Lights: The Novant Health Matthews Medical Center health library works hand in hand with a local organization, SupportWorks, which helps people find, form, and run nonprofit support groups (SupportWorks, 2013). The library refers patrons needing a support group to SupportWorks, and SupportWorks in turn refers patients in need of additional health information to the library.

recreational vehicle designed for that purpose and staffed by nursing personnel. To educate youth in the community about the healthcare profession, the library has provided the Community Care Cruiser with a brochure on this subject, in both English and Spanish.

Community programs are a big part of the services provided by the health library at Novant Health Matthews Medical Center. Aside from health fairs, regularly scheduled outreach programs are held in the community. This gives the library staff a chance to get to know the community it serves before program attendees even know that they may one day need to avail themselves of the library's services. Being visible in the community monthly is a constant reminder of the library's presence.

The medical librarian and library staff work closely with medical center staff to support the needs of patients. A Hispanic man, who spoke only Spanish, came into the emergency department; a recommendation was made for surgery by the physician. Even though emergency department staff was communicating with the patient by way of an interpreter, the patient was reluctant to give his consent for surgery. He wanted to see something in print that described the recommended surgery. The library was called, a printed document detailing the surgery and written in Spanish was provided, and the patient consented to the surgery.

From a patron referral from SupportWorks, the library has developed a long relationship with an African American woman. The woman experiences hypertension, diabetes, and fibromyalgia. Not only has the library provided her with authoritative health information, but they have connected her with resources for free medical assistance in the community. Research by library staff of the medications that the woman was taking identified some duplication of medications. The woman was able to share this information with her physician provider and appropriate changes were made.

The time required to develop a trusting relationship with patients is evidenced in an encounter that the library had with an African American woman who was diagnosed with breast cancer. Many hours were spent with the woman, helping her to understand the treatment options, alleviating her concerns and fears, and finally coming to a place where she was ready to face the difficult months ahead. Following surgery and chemotherapy, the woman called the library one day in tears. She was in the hospital. Medical staff was coming into her room and calling her "mister," unaware that she had lost her hair due to the chemotherapy. She was embarrassed that she had no hair and nothing to cover her head. By this time, the relationship built with library staff was so strong that the woman felt comfortable calling them for help. The medical librarian facilitated obtaining a wig and some head coverings from a local cancer support organization. While certainly not in the usual realm of expectations of a medical librarian, this encounter demonstrates the sensitivity of the librarian to this patient's unique circumstances.

Medical librarians' expanded knowledge of different cultures and ability to locate health information in multiple languages enables them to focus on their patrons' health issues within the context of their ethnicity. As their trust is gained, so is the ability to provide these individuals with the authoritative information they seek to either better understand their health condition or make informed healthcare decisions.

References

Byrd, Darlene (manager of library services, Novant Health Matthews Medical Center) and Shannon Caddell, interview by Donna J. McCloskey, Matthews, North Carolina, August 1, 2013.

Central Intelligence Agency. 2013. *The World Factbook.* https://www.cia.gov/library/publications/the-world-factbook/fields/print_2075.html. Accessed February 24, 2014.

D'Avanzo, CE. 2008. *Pocket Guide to Cultural Health Assessment.* St. Louis, MO: Mosby.

Diller, JV. 2004. *Cultural Diversity: A Primer for the Human Services.* Belmont, CA: Thomson.

Galanti, GA. 2008. *Caring for Patients from Different Cultures.* Philadelphia: University of Pennsylvania Press.

Juckett, G. 2013. "Caring for Latino Patients." *American Family Physician*, 87(1):48–54.

Like, RC, Steiner, RP, and Rubel, AJ. 1996. "Recommended Core Curriculum Guidelines on Culturally Sensitive and Competent Health Care." *Family Medicine*, 28(4):291–97.

Lipson, JG, and Dibble, SL. 2008. *Culture & Clinical Care.* San Francisco: UCSF Nursing Press.

Medical University of South Carolina, College of Medicine. "Cultural Competency." http://etl2.library.musc.edu/cultural/communication/communication_4.php. Accessed January 9, 2013.

Spector, RE. 2013. *Cultural Diversity in Health and Illness.* Upper Saddle River, NJ: Pearson Education.

SupportWorks. 2013. http://www.supportworks.org. Accessed August 2, 2013.

U.S. Census Bureau. 2010. American Fact Finder. "People Reporting Ancestry." http://factfinder2.census.gov. Accessed July 29, 2013.

U.S. Census Bureau. 2012. "US Census Bureau Projections Show a Slower Growing, Older, More Diverse Nation a Half Century from Now." http://www.census.gov/newsroom/releases/archives/population/cb12-243.html. Accessed February 24, 2014.

U.S. Census Bureau. 2013. QuickFacts. "Matthews (town), North Carolina." http://quickfacts.census.gov/qfd/states/37/3741960.html. Accessed August 2, 2013.

U.S. Department of Agriculture. 1986. *Cross-Cultural Counseling: A Guide for Nutrition and Health Counselors.* Washington, DC: U.S. Government Printing Office, 1986. http://archive.org/details/crossculturalcou00usde. Accessed February 24, 2014.

U.S. Department of Health and Human Services, Office of Minority Health, Think Cultural Health. 2013. "National Standards for Culturally and Linguistically Appropriate Services in Health and Health Care." https://www.ThinkCulturalHealth.hhs.gov/Content/clas.asp. Accessed May 6, 2013.

University of Washington Medical Center, Patient and Family Education Services. 2011. *Communication Guide: All Cultures.* Seattle, WA: 2011. http://depts.washington.edu/pfes/PDFs/CommunicationGuideAllCultures.pdf. Accessed February 24, 2014.

12

Marketing Health Library Services to Patients and Consumers

Jackie Davis

HAVING A PASSION FOR THE WORK and role of consumer health librarians will energize the task of marketing those libraries' programs and services. When librarians love what they do, their enthusiasm is contagious. The excitement alone will invite others into the library's world and help the library grow and receive invitations to join the larger efforts of the institution. At a librarian conference a few years ago, a speaker on a marketing panel said the most successful action one can take in the library is to smile. There certainly is more to the story than that, but smiling and passion are a great place to start.

All library work provides the opportunity to serve the surrounding community through a variety of interactions, programs, and information. However, there is something very special about a consumer health library. As mentioned throughout this book, people often come to the library with new diagnoses, fears, and little knowledge of where to turn. The physician may have given the patient good facts and direction (and may have even referred the patient to the library), yet the patient may not be able to access the information because of language barriers, inability to read the material, unfamiliarity with medical vocabulary, or simply because anxiety may interfere with the ability to hear and absorb the physician's explanations and next steps. Without some ability to understand their diagnosis, patients and family members cannot participate in their self-care, make treatment choices based on solid data, fully comply with medical instructions, and advocate for themselves within the complex structures of today's healthcare system.

This inability to understand and make sense of healthcare information has been discussed in this book as health literacy. Health literacy not only affects patients' ability to participate in their treatment, but also is a very large drain on the national economy. As reported by Vernon, "The savings that could be achieved by improving health literacy—a lower bound of $106 billion and an upper bound of $238 billion—translate into enough funds to insure every one of the more than 47 million persons who lacked coverage in the United States in 2006" (Vernon, 2007). Lilian Hill, who writes about health education and literacy makes a further point,

> The highly educated will usually find their way to the knowledge they need and have the skills to navigate the healthcare system to get the answers they want. However, the health outcomes for others may be very different. As adult educa-tors we express concern for the poor and underprivileged among us and many of us espouse a belief in social action; this is an arena where I believe our critical engagement is warranted. (Hill, 2007)

The consumer health librarian has the very special opportunity to make information accessible and understandable with the resources he or she has available. It is an exciting and humbling role.

Seeing patient education as a social justice imperative fuels a passion for the work involved. There are multiple aspects to the concept of social justice, but this chapter explores two in particular: (1) inclusion of everyone in the full benefits of society and (2) empowerment of people to participate fully in the economic, social, and cultural life of the country, as defined by the Institute for Intellectual Property & Social Justice on its website (Institute for Intellec-tual Property & Social Justice, Inc., 2003). It is appropriate to add to the list "to participate fully in one's medical decisions." No longer can consumers of health walk into the doctor's office and passively say, "Make me well." In fact, more physicians are asking their patients to participate and make decisions about how they will be treated (Say, 2003). Without resources for educating oneself about the options and for learning good preventive health measures, there cannot be shared empowerment of health consumers.

There is no one solution at this time for these pressing consumer health lit-eracy issues so critical to patient care. Ganz says, positioning the library to be able to meet these informational needs "is to figure out how to break through the inertia of habit to get people to pay attention" (Ganz, 2009). When the li-brarian takes an avid focus on health literacy, and applies a creative energy in seeking resources and methods for delivering health information, the library becomes a powerful place to enact social change.

There are two primary constituencies with which health librarians engage: the community and the healthcare institution. There are important messages about the library and different ways to convey them to each group. Within the hospital, the library can promote the belief that every healthcare worker is responsible for making health and medical information understandable to patients. The second message is the supportive role the library can play in meeting this responsibility. Community messages identify the library as a resource for good health information in a variety of formats. Additionally, there are locale-specific and larger community needs that the library may want to address. Some health libraries focus on providing excellent community programming; others conduct outreach to a variety of organizations. Speaking in the community and participating in area health fairs is an important component of working with the local population. It's often an enjoyable way to build outside relationships while teaching people specific ways to be good health information consumers.

More recently there have been discussions about the limits of "educating" patients and the value of "engaging" patients in their learning. Dr. Mike Evans, a family physician and a self-proclaimed re-inventor of patient education, says on his website, http://www.myfavouritemedicine.com/, that stories trump data, and relationships trump stories (Evans, 2013). The staff in the consumer health library provide education (data) and in the course of the brief encounter, *engage* the customer through listening and professional compassion. The connection between the library staff and the patients/families/community members personalizes learning and helps connect the consumer with information in a warm, caring way. It is the sensitivity and kindness of the staff that assists in creating the ever-so-valuable personal story, and thus the data become meaningful in the context of the relationship. Each encounter with a patient or customer is an opportunity to demonstrate that the library is a safe, welcoming place where customers are encouraged to return and share their experience with others.

Health Information Ambassador

Depending on the hospital setting, health libraries are often hidden or in another building altogether. Libraries need emissaries and advocates at all levels of the organization. Staff also needs to understand they can call on the librarian to provide evidence-based patient health or medical information and have it delivered to the patient's room, if needed.

Marketing the Library

Marketing is the entire effort to connect the consumer with the product and keep the customer coming back for more. Marketing is not a one-time

Bright Lights: A hospital-based program that has received attention recently, and is a great example of creating relationships and connections as well as stories, is the Health Ambassador for the Patient Education program at Sharp Memorial Hospital in San Diego, California. This program is a partnership with the Volunteer Department where the volunteers conduct patient rounds and ask the patients or their family members if they would like to have any further information about their health concerns. The volunteers write requests on an intake form and bring it to the health librarian, who researches and prints the articles; volunteers return to the patient's room with the material. This activity has been a success primarily because the volunteer has the time to listen to the patient, expressing interest and compassion. It is the personalized engagement in the context of patient education which brings an inestimable value to the "data" (Davis, 2013). The Ambassadors take the services of the library out to where they are needed. In doing so, they also provide consistent publicity about the library to staff on the patient care units.

campaign, or one particular vehicle. It requires the long view with consistent actions to continually remind people that the consumer health library is their go-to resource for high-quality, trusted, personalized, and caring information. Much of what has been written about marketing for libraries has been adapted from the business world, with a focus on products or services for paying customers. Libraries can learn much from tested and proven marketing strategies.

However, the library's marketing strategy emphasizes a *story* rather than a product. This narrative must describe the value of the library, staff, materials, and programs. As mentioned previously, there is a constant need for the library to make successful connections between its resources and services to patients, consumers, community members, and professional healthcare providers. Kathy Dempsey writes in her book, *The Accidental Library Marketer* (Dempsey, 2009), that most libraries look at marketing tasks as another "duty as assigned" rather than prioritizing and embedding them in an overall library plan. In many instances, the need for marketing arises when a program is scheduled or a new service is provided. Without an overall marketing plan for informing others, often a staff member "accidentally" finds him- or herself in the position of creating a flyer or a website announcement. If the librarian does a good job, the next person who plans a library event will ask him or her to create a new announcement and, in this haphazard way, eventually this staff person assumes charge of library marketing.

In this era of shrinking health library budgets (and shrinking and disappearing healthcare libraries), it is imperative that librarians and staff make sure others know the significance of the library and its value to the organization. In order to do this well, marketing cannot be just a flyer or announcement. Library staff know the importance of their work as they connect daily with grateful patients and the public. Statements from staff and patients such as, "I didn't know you were here" can be disheartening. These statements may also serve as an incentive to review the library's marketing efforts. The goal is to develop creative new strategies for the library to further the hospital's overall mission, thus securing its essential role in the organization and community at large.

Creating the Plan

In creating a plan, Dempsey (http://www.LibrariesAreEssential.com) separates the various tasks of marketing, and clarifies terms that are often used synonymously but inaccurately:

- **Marketing** is taking steps to move goods from producers to consumers. It's determining what people want, delivering it, evaluating consumer satisfaction, and then periodically updating the whole process.
- **Public relations** is a planned, long-term communication program (via various media) with a goal of helping people to think well of an organization, product, or concept.
- **Publicity** is sending a message via official channels such as new releases, newsletters, and press conferences.
- **Promotion** is furthering the growth or development of a product or service. It's not just aiming towards good will; it is encouraging people to use that product or service by telling people how it benefits them.
- **Advertising** is calling attention to something through paid announcements.
- **Branding** has dual objectives: (1) establishing a strong link between a company and its logo/typeface/picture or name/phrase, and (2) developing the "personality" of a product or service by establishing the characteristics that should come to mind when people think of it. Branding helps build loyalty.
- **Advocacy** is getting people who have good opinions of an organization to speak to others on its behalf, to convince other people of its value (Dempsey, 2009).

Addressing each one of these activities results in a marketing plan the library develops and implements, in some form and to some extent, daily. As each category is part of a whole, each can be looked at separately. Dempsey says marketing in the business world is about moving goods, and in libraries it is about services, programs, and materials. However, she points out that marketing is also the assessment of the library's services and programs, through surveys and other tools. Additionally, she recommends doing these assessments in a structured way, on a regular basis, for a continual look at what the library has to offer.

Strategies

The following from Dempsey's list of marketing tasks may be handled through the corporate marketing or business department: *public relations*, *publicity*, and *paid advertising*. To begin, request a meeting to discuss the library's events and how best to coordinate for publicity and advertising. Which tasks may the library manage on its own? Suggest special library services that can be highlighted in corporate public relations efforts. Submit press releases to announce library activities or honors. News outlets usually have a health reporter who can be cultivated for media coverage. News media may request the information in a particular format, and often want to highlight activities that correspond with the news of the day or the health theme of the month (e.g., Breast Cancer Month is October).

Additional avenues for *advertising and promotional* activities may have costs associated even if they don't take the form of paid print space or radio airtime. Printing a quarterly newsletter lets customers know about new items available for borrowing, programs or events, consumer health websites, and other information that advertises the library's value. One way to create the mailing list is through opt-in sign-up sheets at community health fairs and by including it on the library's form filled out by new cardholders. Ask for preferred delivery methods. The newsletter, and other information, can be saved in PDF or other electronic format, then sent out through email. It can also be printed and sent through the post office. Consider adding others to the library's mailing list such as local public libraries, any other medical libraries, other health agencies, elected officials, and specific departments in local colleges and universities. The library may want to send out holiday cards or holiday e-greetings each year. The human connection and goodwill generated by this seemingly small act will reinforce the library's friendships and supporters.

There are other printed materials that can be developed and distributed both within the hospital and in the community to advertise the library, such as business cards, bookmarks, and library labels put on educational pamphlets. That said, many people will turn to the hospital's website to learn more about the library and possibly use it as a portal for additional quality

Internet health information resources. The library's website should be carefully evaluated for clarity, quantity and quality of information, currency, and, most importantly, to ensure the message the staff wants to convey is actually expressed through its website content. Share library contact information with users and also have the catalog accessible online. Explore the potential value of making the website available through a mobile device. A good measure for gauging the quality of the site is to garner the user's perspective. Conducting usability testing and user surveys will make for a much better product because it is the user who will help illuminate areas that could be improved.

As mentioned in Chapter 9, the avenues into social media and networking websites may be structured or restricted through the corporate marketing department. If hospital policy allows a presence on Facebook, Yelp, Twitter, YouTube, blog site, etc., these are excellent ways to communicate the who, what, where, and why of the library and to engage with the participating community as long as there is a commitment to keep up the conversation in a timely way. With the rise of social media, users are more aware and sensitive to privacy concerns, and this needs to be addressed clearly if the library chooses to promote on social media sites.

Branding is a critical task that positions the library as *the* resource for relevant and quality consumer health information in a professional and compassionate setting. It is the story of the library that is told in every vehicle of communication. Dempsey writes that there are two facets to branding. It includes all the visual cues on printed materials, perhaps including a slogan, as well as signage. Each piece of material that leaves the library should be labeled and include the library's contact information. If letters, pathfinders, or flyers are developed, these should have a consistent logo, color, and typeface. However, this is only a slice of the task and the simpler facet of branding. Dempsey refers to the additional piece as creating and maintaining a "personality." It requires some structured conversation with the staff and is covered further in the following section called "Creating Your Story."

The area of *advocacy*, getting others to spread the word about the library, is an exciting way to see the fruits of the library's labors in action. Once staff, patients, and community members discover the library's ability to empower individuals, many will share this good news. Librarians can bring their expertise to committees working towards a healthier community as another way to advocate for their profession as well as their library's assets. There may be a local task force that is moving health literacy issues forward; the librarian's participation in these efforts as a subject expert is yet another way to advocate for those who are marginalized in the healthcare system. It is rewarding to align the work of the library and hospital with the efforts of other community leaders who appreciate the critical importance of informed health consumers.

Community Organizing

Many librarians have already been working with business marketing and outreach models adapted for the library setting and have developed their own resourceful ideas for "getting the word out." There's an additional model that helps the library create and sustain a climate that supports patient education and engagement. Known as community organizing, it utilizes some of the best of the marketing approach and integrates these ideas into an overall approach. This is where advocacy, about which Dempsey writes in her list of marketing activities, can come into powerful focus. Community organizing is often associated with political and social movements to empower groups of people. However, aspects of community organizing can add spark and creativity to guide health libraries' work within their institutions. In a nutshell, community organizing is all about strong *relationship building*—for an altruistic purpose. Unlike the business marketing approach, this model assumes:

- A belief in the moral imperative of providing accessible consumer health resources, empowering patients to advocate for themselves within the healthcare system.
- Staff of the hospital, and the surrounding community-at-large, will benefit from the library's quality health resources and the librarian's valuable services.
- The hospital's goals are to provide the highest quality of care to the greatest number of people, which requires informed patients who can make the best decisions with their healthcare providers.

Reframing and seeing the library's work as a catalyst for social justice in healthcare can drive the passion and direction of its marketing strategies. Different from simple public relations, community organizing is about building relationships and influencing a culture shift—in this case, embracing patient information, education, and empowerment as vital to patient care. Community organizing positions the library as "the right thing" for patients and the community. Through a shared passion, others strongly enlist in the library's efforts to educate the consumer, to understand and work on the issues of health literacy, and effectively inform leaders of the library's important role in meeting the hospital's mission. Using community organizing as the framework for creating a library action plan changes marketing's role from a business model to one of social betterment.

Debra Askanase, who calls herself an Engagement Strategist on her blog *Community Organizer 2.0*, posted a visual model, which she adapted from Seth Godin's "The Circles of Marketing." This model demonstrates how the

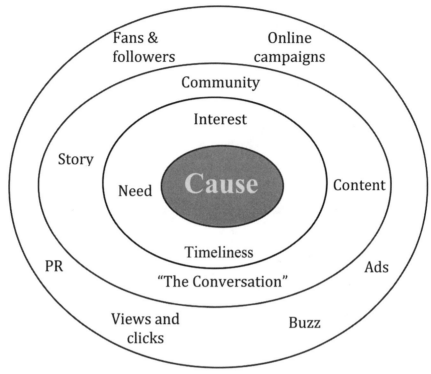

FIGURE 12.1
The Circles of Nonprofit Marketing

tasks of marketing would align if they were motivated by a social cause with community organizing as the framework (Askanase, 2012).

The author observes that the outer circle, where marketing takes place, is the final aspect of the work, and the second circle is the part of the plan where community building takes place. It's in the second circle where the library's story is created with staff, customers, and hospital personnel, and where "The Conversation" occurs about the value of providing health information as a way to empower patients, loved ones, and those who are trying to stay well. This message of empowerment emphasizes the importance of providing health information in the hospital and throughout the community.

Libraries need others to embrace the story and become passionate about services such as addressing health literacy. The second circle focuses on how to develop relationships; create allies with like-minded hospital leaders; enlist, mobilize, and join with established support networks; and launch a campaign that embeds the library as part of the hospital's core mission. Like a domino effect, those structural or institutional relationships will then carry the library's compelling message onward. It is a real success to have others bring the library's story forward, telling patients and families to visit the library or calling the librarian to have information brought to the patient's room. This shared passion for patient information as a form of empowerment guides the work ahead.

Marshall Ganz has written extensively about community organizing. He says organizing is most effective at creating change when an organization tells its story. In marketing parlance, this might be called the elevator speech, but in this context, the story is richer and more powerful. If the library is to lead, it has to know its story. There is the historical story of the library, of course. More captivating are the daily efforts, patient by patient, of acquiring meaningful health information, teaching patients how to make sense of the healthcare system, and be better healthcare consumers. Ganz further states that once a story is told, the moral is not simply a concept but a statement from the heart.

> If you don't interpret to others your calling and your reason for doing what you're doing, do you think it will just stay uninterpreted? No. Other people will interpret it for you. You don't have any choice if you want to be a leader. You have to claim authorship of your story and learn to tell it to others so they can understand the values that move you to act, because it might move them to act as well. (Ganz, 2009)

Creating and sharing this story among library staff is the beginning of building an "us," a motivated team sharing a similar fervor for the library's work and its goals. Sharing it beyond the library is the beginning of forging stronger community relationships.

Creating the Story (or Branding a Personality)

The library's story is constructed through individual staff sharing: what moves them to come to work every morning? What customer concerns did they solve? And why is it critical to give patients tools of empowerment? Identifying these individual stories and then examining them for common themes will help the library construct its unique narrative. Elisabeth Doucett further describes the story as

> the articulation of the role it plays or wants to play in its community. To create a powerful story, the library needs to identify a role that no one else can duplicate. The story is meant to inform anyone considering using the library about what makes it special and worth visiting. (Doucett, 2008)

For instance, the story may be that the library is *the* source of consumer health information for patients and families. It may describe a warm and welcoming place, where no one leaves empty handed. The story might weave in special services such as how the librarian brings information to the patient's bedside. The library's users should share their experiences, too. The goal is to create relationships and stories that become the pathway to changing minds and moving hearts. Doucett points out, "A meaningful story will motivate potential patrons to come to the library because they are seeking what the library provides" (Doucett, 2008). Additionally, a powerful story will motivate the hospital staff to think first of the library as a resource for their patients.

Assessing the Library

The next step is an assessment of the library's services, programs, collections, communication strategies, and physical facility. Chapter 2 offers an in-depth guide for conducting any type of library assessment including the SWOT (*s*trengths, *w*eaknesses, *o*pportunities, and *t*hreats) analysis. This is an effective way to identify relevant issues and inform the work ahead. Dempsey suggests using the SWOT analysis after doing a customer survey, as well as using staff input (Dempsey, 2009). Some questions to begin this assessment:

- Is the guiding principle of patient empowerment and self-advocacy at the forefront of the workday?
- What services does the library offer, and which are valued by the customers? These questions can be answered by both the quantitative (statistics) and qualitative (stories, quotes) data gathered over time. Surveys would be an additional resource for the SWOT analysis.
- What services do staff value but are not well used? Why keep them?
- What needs to be publicized more? Do these activities align with the values of justice and accessibility?
- How do others learn about new items, services, or programs? Who are the intended recipients of the services? Who is missing from the picture?
- Who are the best supporters and champions of the library, in and out of the hospital?
- Which committees do staff attend and how do staff bring value to each one? How do they communicate about the library?
- Who are the regular customers and why do they return?
- Are the procedures for check-out, reference requests, or resources user-friendly?

- Is the website user-friendly and up to date? Are other social media being used effectively?

As stated earlier, the library's physical facility should factor into the SWOT analysis. A patient who just received an alarming diagnosis should feel as if the library is a safe place to get information. An atmosphere of tidy organization is more inviting than one that communicates confusion, which could easily send an anxious patient away. Identify exactly what aspects of the physical facility customers like (e.g., smells, colors, art, water fountain, etc.). Although libraries are getting away from the "shushing" stereotype, it is still important that the consumer health library be quiet, relaxing, and private.

There is a concept called "inbound marketing" that focuses on *earning* the interest of the customer instead of *buying* it. From a library perspective, this requires making the website, newsletter, and emails so valuable that those vehicles draw customers *into* the library (Drell, 2011). When customers arrive, they deserve a place that expresses self-empowerment through a wide range of resources offered by a caring staff.

Supporting customers through relevant, useful information becomes a positive experience they will convey to others. Staff attitudes also need to be included in the analysis. Everyone has strengths to offer in this effort; the abilities and interests of each person add depth to the library's services and story.

Time for Action

One final phase of the analysis is to reference the organization's five-year strategic plan to ensure the alignment of the library's mission with the institution's priorities. Identify organizational needs the library can support. Maybe the organization has a patient education team and the library can participate or at least be a resource. Many hospitals focus on patient-/family-centered care, and one of the core tenets of this philosophy is patient education. The library's services *can* fill some gaps, promoting the issues of health literacy and consumer education, while gaining new supporters in the process. The aspirations of the library are best served when the interests of the hospital and community are served; this requires thorough analysis based upon solid data.

Finally, the organizational action planning requires outreach to the larger community. Grassroots organizing is a natural, organic way of connecting people with ideas. However, in order for the natural flow of connection to begin, the librarian has to get out of the library and meet with the "folks." The folks in this situation are the hospital and community leaders, the influencers who support patient education and empowerment. These are the people who will enable organizational plans to unfold.

In reaching out to these individuals, several important messages must remain constant. The first is that the library staff wants to be proactive in supporting the work of organizational leaders and committees dedicated to patient information, patient education, health literacy, and patient empowerment. The additional but critical piece is that the library is aligned with the overall goals of the hospital's brand and focus. Ask how the library can be of service to institutional leadership; invite suggestions for library materials and recommendations. Some healthcare providers may never come into the library unless they are invited, so making the invitation personal is important. Call the managers, or walk up to their offices and meet them. Make librarian rounds on the staff and smile. Have the library's story ready to share off the top of your head. Send stories to the administration and share them at committee meetings. It is through slow, steady relationship-building that people are won over, thus becoming the biggest supporters and marketers for the library.

Take the same approach to engaging community connections. Send letters to area senior services, health agencies and organizations, community service clubs, support groups, health fair organizers, etc., and let them know a health librarian is available to speak at their events. See if there is a speakers' bureau in the county health organization and ask to be added to their list. Connect by phone or letter with the local public health schools, local nursing schools, and high school health, physical education, and science teachers. Let people know the librarian can speak with their church or service groups. As word travels, the community will invite the librarian to events and to participate in health initiatives.

Conclusion

Consumer health libraries have an important mission as evidenced by patients who arrive beset by doubts and leave with new confidence, equipped with information and referrals to additional resources. There are people who haven't grasped the concept of being a healthcare consumer, yet upon understanding its implications say that they wished they had learned earlier about the consumer health library. To achieve its mission, the library must rethink how it connects with the healthcare profession, patients, and consumers. Community organizing is a creative and effective way to firmly establish the library in the hospital and geographic locale, ensuring its place as the established go-to resource for consumer health information.

References

Askanase, D. 2012. "The Circles of Non-Profit Marketing." *CommunityOrganizer2.0.* http://communityorganizer20.com/2012/08/09/the-circles-of-nonprofit-marketing. Accessed August 9, 2013.

Davis, J. 2013. "Health Information Ambassador Program for Patient Education: A Best Practice for Bringing the Consumer Health Library to the Patient." *Journal of Consumer Health on the Internet*, 17(1):25–34.

Dempsey, K. 2009. *The Accidental Library Marketer.* Medford, NJ: Information Today, Inc.

Doucett, E. 2008. *Creating Your Library Brand: Communicating Your Relevance and Value to Your Patrons.* Chicago: American Library Association.

Drell, L. 2011. "Inbound-Outbound-Marketing." Mashable. October 30, 2011. http://mashable.com/2011/10/30/inbound-outbound-marketing. Accessed August 31, 2013.

Evans, M. 2013. "Top 8 Talk Handout," My Favourite Medicine. April 2013. http://www.myfavouritemedicine.com/wp-content/uploads/2013/04/Evans-Top-8-Talk-Hand-Out.pdf. Accessed August 31, 2013.

Ganz, M. 2009. "Why Stories Matter: The Art and Craft of Social Change." *Sojourners.* March 2009. http://sojo.net/magazine/2009/03/why-stories-matter. Accessed August 31, 2013.

Hill, LH. 2007. "Health Literacy as a Social Justice Issue that Affects Us All." Literacy Information and Communication System. June 5, 2007. http://lincs.ed.gov/piper mail/diversity/2007/000788.html. Accessed August 24, 2013.

Institute for Intellectual Property & Social Justice, Inc. 2003. "Social Justice Definition." http://www.iipsj.org/index.php?option=com_content&view=article&id=25 &Itemid=30. Accessed August 24, 2013.

Say, R. 2003. "The Importance of Patient Preference in Treatment Decisions—Challenges for Doctors." *BMJ*, 327(7414):542–45.

Vernon, JA. 2007. "Low Health Literacy: Implications for National Health Policy." George Washington University. October 4, 2007. http://hsrc.himmelfarb.gwu.edu/ sphhs_policy_facpubs/index.3.html. Accessed February 24, 2014.

13

Strategic Partnerships

Carol Ann Attwood

Overview of Collaboration for Strategic Partnerships

CONSUMER HEALTH LIBRARIES AND librarians have long shown innovation in searching out collaborations and alliances internally within their organizational structures and also in making connections externally that would benefit not only the library and its functions but also the communities in which they reside. In this section, we will review the importance of strategic alliances and collaborations that benefit not only consumers but also the libraries and communities that libraries serve. As discussed in Chapter 12, the principles of community organizing are applicable in forming these important alliances.

As with most organizations, consumer health libraries also have mission statements that optimally are in sync with the organization's strategic objectives. Mission statements have been characteristically described as "a clear and concise summary of your library's unique contribution to your organization's success" (American Association of Law Librarians, 2013), but in order for a mission statement to be successful all members of the library team must embrace the values that it outlines. A mission statement without accompanying strategic objectives is meaningless. In turn, lack of strategic objectives impacts the services provided and, ultimately, the ways in which the consumer health library effectively serves the needs of its patrons. Strategic objectives often include forming and maintaining purposeful partnerships. These partnerships are characterized by two organizations or departments working together symbiotically towards a common goal. Such relationships can be used constructively in the current healthcare market by bringing the best practices of each department together to optimize resources and enlarge the reach of each one's individual programming. As noted by Murray in *The Wall Street Journal Essential Guide to Management* (Murray, 2010), "In the end, strategy and execution must become . . . one and the same." In difficult financial times for healthcare organizations, this concept becomes paramount; a firm strategy is vital to foster and maintain partnerships that will evolve, flourish, and continue to serve as a stepping stone for new initiatives.

Much is written in the business literature on the importance of strategic partnerships, which consumer health librarians can extrapolate to build their own. As consumer health librarians review their roles in light of the strategic objectives of the organization, they can better align themselves in a way that emphasizes their unique role in meeting those stated goals. In addition to organizational strategic objectives, librarians must also understand the larger workplace culture. Organizational culture is described not only in terms of workplace culture but also in the importance of the silent political forces that drive the culture and values of an organization (Koerner and Wesley, 2008). The book, *The Five Most Important Questions You Will Ever Ask about Your Organization* (Drucker, 2008), focuses on organizational self-assessment utilizing five key questions: (1) What is the mission? (2) Who is the customer? (3) What does the customer value? (4) What are the results? and (5) What is the plan? Answering these questions can assist the consumer health librarian in focusing on both department-specific goals as well as the strategic objectives of the organization-at-large.

In today's marketplace, consumer health librarians must be able to clearly articulate how the services provided are tightly linked to the objectives of the organization and must use every opportunity to share that linkage through communication with peers, consumers, administrators, and decision-makers. Becoming a visual presence outside of the confines of the consumer health library walls is a vital first step that librarians must take. Doing so enhances their visibility and puts them in a position to influence policy-makers about the importance of the library's services. The positive effects of collaboration and strategic partnerships are many, including an increased profile, the opportunity to showcase programming offered, the linkages between services and the primary objectives of the organization, and the positive good will that communicating and interacting with others within the organization can provide both in the present and for future initiatives. Through showcasing organizational collaborations that have been established and then building upon those relationships, a springboard is developed from which to launch services and programming into the greater community.

Throughout healthcare, there is diminishing funding for services that do not provide a positive return on investment. The wise consumer health librarian is aware of the impact current changes in healthcare delivery bring to the organization as well as to patients and consumers. Currently, accountable care, which emphasizes quality and positive outcomes, is front and center as the Affordable Care Act takes effect (U.S. Department of Health and Human Services, 2013). Consumer health librarians are uniquely poised to provide services around the many aspects of the Affordable Care Act and can help healthcare organizations address the needs of patient empowerment and engagement through access to information and educational materials. It is incumbent upon consumer health librarians to educate organizational decision-makers on the role they can play in self-empowerment as a means to develop patients' and consumers' ability to embrace healthier lifestyles and to better care for their chronic healthcare concerns.

Best Practices for Strategic Partnerships and Collaboration

The following pages outline examples of how consumer health librarians might embed themselves into the fiber of healthcare reform, healthcare delivery, and the provision of information and services that will optimize the patient experience. The practices work to place the consumer health library at the center of change and demonstrate improved healthcare outcomes.

The Joint Commission, a healthcare accreditation body that promulgates standards for hospitals and health organizations to provide safe and effective care while maintaining quality and managing costs (Joint Commission, 2013), has placed patient safety at the heart of its certification requirements. One way to address this need is for the consumer health library to collaborate with their organization's quality or risk management team to initiate a service providing written or electronic information to at-risk-for-falls patients that outlines strategies to avoid falls while in the hospital or after discharge. Gathering best practices tips from professional interdisciplinary groups provide the background for consumer health librarians to work collaboratively with quality or risk management and patient educators, developing needed brochures and handouts to share with patients and their providers.

A core function of healthcare organizations and, correspondingly, consumer health libraries is health promotion and wellness initiatives. Whether collaboration occurs within the organization through workplace wellness program or outside of the library to the community-at-large, there are many ways to optimize these opportunities. Approaches the consumer health librarian can take to be included as an integral part of internal workplace wellness initiatives include serving on multidisciplinary teams, offering Lunch and Learn sessions on health and wellness topics, hosting workplace wellness groups (e.g., Weight Watchers), or providing one-on-one assistance with helpful, relevant consumer health apps on mobile devices. Other ideas include using information from the Pew Internet and Family Life Project surveys (Pew Research Center, 2013) to highlight current research findings and inform healthcare employees or members of the general public on how to retrieve quality Internet information on these topics. In addition, the consumer health librarian might offer to write articles for a recurring health promotion column in the employee newsletter. Short snippets of information (e.g., Health Bytes) would offer employees the opportunity to further explore selected healthcare topics. If the organization has classes on weight manage-ment, desk stretches, or yoga classes, classroom space in the consumer health library might be repurposed to offer these classes. Doing so highlights the library's other services for employees and their family members and allows for simultaneous marketing.

These collaborations demonstrate programs that the healthcare organiza-tion can also promote in the community through public libraries, community or senior centers, or faith-based centers. Often, resources for community programming are at a premium, so reaching out and offering tested program-ming while marketing the library's and parent organization's services benefits all. Partnering with public librarians builds relationships that may lead to other opportunities (e.g., training opportunities for health resources offered by the consumer health librarian in the public library). In addition to public libraries, consumer health librarians can reach out to senior centers, public health departments, and others to co-sponsor programs on immunizations prior to the start of school, offer active aging resources for the aged fifty and up population, provide health information resources for those who are not English speaking, and also provide resources for those with health literacy needs. These strategic alliances can be strengthened with dual marketing at community health fairs or other community events, thus pointing consumers in the right direction to meet their health information needs.

Several programs have been successfully developed on the topics noted previously (e.g., the National Library of Medicine/National Institutes of Health's "Helping Older Adults Search for Health Information Online: A Toolkit for Trainers," [http://nihseniorhealth.gov/toolkit/toolkit.html]). This five-session tutorial with lesson plans and sample searches helps librarians train older adults how to optimize their online health information searches. Such a course could be offered anywhere—the consumer health library or a community location—with the modules co-taught by the consumer health and public health librarians. Offering this course could be an ongoing collaboration between public and consumer health librarians and serve as a portal for enhanced programming on senior and other healthcare topics.

As mentioned at the beginning of this chapter, an important approach is to review the organization's strategic objectives, including any initiatives that are priorities for the next five years. Determine what information or educational needs patients, their family members, and healthcare providers will need for the organization to realize these priorities then develop collaborative complementary programs to address them.

> **Bright Lights:** At a comprehensive cancer center, a strategic priority was to focus on patient education and health information. A collaborative relationship between a consumer health library and the American Cancer Society (ACS) Navigator was forged (Attwood and Wellik, 2012). The consumer health library housed the office of the ACS Navigator, as well as the classroom where classes on chemotherapy and nutrition during cancer therapy were held. This collaboration allowed current cancer patients and their family members to see the many resources the consumer health library had to offer, including consumer health and medical textbooks, cancer journals and newsletters, brochures, booklets, and models, as well as cancer pathfinders on the library's website. In addition, cancer center visitors to the library could be directed to the many classes and support services provided by the ACS Navigator, including prosthesis, wigs, accommodations, travel allocations, and support groups. With this collaboration, other professionals were drawn into the library activities such as the cancer nurse patient education specialist as well as the chemotherapy and radiation therapy care team members who then, based upon their familiarity with the library staff, directed patients to the library and its services.

There is no end to the number of departments or groups the consumer health librarian can work with to help meet patients' health information needs. In this author's organization, a strategic partnership with transplant services provided brochures and links on the consumer health website that optimized information even as patients awaited transplants. Using the collective knowledge and expertise of the transplant team, the consumer health library built a catalog of resources to share with patients, family members, and potential donors.

Another potential collaboration is highlighted by the Patient Protection and Affordable Care Act, regarding the prevention of thirty-day readmissions. Stone and Hoffman (2010) noted linkages can be made with care managers and patients to encourage compliance with discharge instructions. This provides an opportunity for the consumer health library to serve as an additional information portal for recently discharged patients, complementing other discharge information, and encouraging patients' self-help behavior and family support. Such informed self-determination helps reduce thirty-day readmission rates. It also responds to Medicare reimbursement policies, which often preclude payment when patients are readmitted within thirty days of discharge for the same diagnosis.

Consumer health librarians may also market their resources internally by speaking to staff and other healthcare providers at unit meetings, supervisory meetings, and physicians' grand rounds, especially to discuss new resources and to highlight virtual search capabilities for providers. An example of this type of collaboration could be with physicians whose patients have chronic healthcare conditions like fibromyalgia. The consumer health library could develop virtual, specialized information packets for these patients that would include material on coping mechanisms and links to new research and treatment options by featuring resources provided by the healthcare organization or from clinical trials' websites. This would allow the patient and family to search and find new research that may be of benefit to them and which they can share and discuss with their healthcare providers.

Many healthcare organizations now provide secure, virtual access for patients to view their medical records, appointments, problem lists, current medications, clinical notes, and allergies at any time. This can also be an avenue for consumer health librarians, working with web developers to attach pertinent resource links. New electronic health records may also have this function, allowing the provider to print information from preselected health information databases at the point of care.

Partnerships and strategic alliances between the consumer health librarian and patients and family may also be fostered through a consumer health website that can be viewed by hospitalized patients. For minimal costs, a patient portal can be developed with a laptop computer or smart device that will allow the patient to access specific pathfinders on health topics and hospital resources. Also, the consumer health library can provide printed or virtual information on how to be a cyber-savvy searcher, filtering out those healthcare resources that are not authoritative, those offering miracle cures, or seeking to sell healthcare products to unsuspecting consumers. With the advent of electronic resources and targeting those who are using social media for many transactions of daily living, the consumer health librarian can develop specific social media sites on YouTube, Facebook, or Twitter, or connect the consumer to specific blogs and podcasts that have been developed by providers within the organization. Optimizing social media sites could work in tandem with print-focused resources for those without immediate access to computer networks.

To help meet the education and information needs of patients with low health literacy, the librarian can partner with patient educators, nurses, and other healthcare professionals to provide information with illustrations or other easy-to-read options. The National Library of Medicine's consumer health website, MedlinePlus, provides many online tutorials with illustrations that would assist those who have difficulties reading or understanding medical terminology. These tutorials can be used repeatedly to help patients assimilate information on self-care and learn when to seek additional assistance from their providers. Another avenue to explore is the relationship between the consumer health library and the internal hospital community. Highlighting the functions of the consumer health library not only externally to consumers, patients, and family members, but also internally to hospital employees is strategically important. Hospital staff can be the most effective marketing agents for the consumer health library, as word of mouth carries far beyond the library itself. By describing library resources to employee groups such as nurses (who typically comprise the largest number of healthcare workers in a given organization), the consumer health librarian can build effective alliances, as library resources will help nurses make more efficient use of their time in educating patients about their diseases and how to deal with chronic symptoms. An astute consumer health librarian constantly interviews and communicates with a variety of healthcare workers to learn about upcoming initiatives, meanwhile selecting library resources to bring forward as new programs are being planned. As mentioned previously, the consumer health librarian needs to move beyond the walls of the library and will need to serve as the primary marketing tool and innovator for programming, which can be as diverse as offering space for computer-based classes to creating graphics to assist others in displaying their program ideas within and outside the organization.

If the healthcare organization has a research focus, the consumer health librarian can post a list of topical, peer-reviewed articles from medical journals that can be shared on the library's website or presented in forums such as executive councils, clinical staff meetings, or health promotion committees. Research is constantly being updated, and the librarian can be the key person to disseminate this information. The librarian can also provide additional resources to meet strategic objectives on issues as diverse as accessibility to care, resource management, medical home models, or accountable care organizations.

Community outreach can be structured in several ways, all informed by an assessment of community needs. Nonprofit healthcare organizations are required by provisions in the Affordable Care Act to perform a community needs assessment every three years to retain their 501(c)(3) status (Internal Revenue Service, 2013). Using the hospital's most current community needs assessment can help inform partnership opportunities for the consumer health librarian. Potential partnerships include those with public health departments, area agencies on aging, veterans' resources, public school systems, public libraries, and faith-based centers. An example is to align consumer health library resources with military and governmental agencies, such as Wounded Warriors, in which the consumer health librarian develops pathfinders on depression, post-traumatic stress disorder, traumatic brain injury, and the like. The librarian can also offer veterans and their families a central location within the library for their support groups and for locating resources in skills training, housing, and other community-based services.

In today's world of accountable care organizations, healthcare reform, quality outcomes, and changing reimbursement, the consumer health librarian can assist healthcare decision-makers in finding targeted evidence from peer-reviewed medical journals to promote and substantiate decision-making on organizational programming and services. The consumer health librarian is uniquely qualified to produce a substantive, systematic review and can define search strategies by journal, publication date, or tiered research findings. These skills place the librarian in the center of the decision-making process, further highlighting the visibility and varied functions of the consumer health library.

Another external alliance is to conduct work with case or continuing care managers at the hospital, its ambulatory care clinics and assisted living facilities, with the goal of providing their patients relevant, readable healthcare information on a variety of topics. A system can be devised for the librarian to interview patients who would benefit most from this service. Healthcare reforms focusing on continuing care management is a launching point for librarians to share their expertise, accessing information that improves patient care and lowers healthcare costs by empowering patients to take charge of their care outcomes. This patient-focused care model can be replicated among healthcare organizations and providers to focus on population health management strategies that keep individuals as healthy as possible, while also encouraging them to take responsibility for their healthcare behaviors. Website links to healthcare reform information, accountable care organizations, Medicare/Medicaid, Social Security Disability, and any number of other supporting organizations can help to build alliances while keeping consumers in contact with the most up-to-date information on applying for benefits, important regulatory requirements, and changes in healthcare delivery systems.

Creating a consumer health library kiosk is another outreach approach to patients, their family members, and providers. These can be either standalone centers or desks with laptops or tabletop computers, keyboards, and printers. The consumer health librarian can market these resources within their organization as well as in the community-at-large and can populate them with social media resources such as the organization's Facebook, Twitter, or YouTube pages, along with podcasts, blogs, patient portals, and links to pathfinders on reliable, relevant websites and portable health apps. Upkeep of the kiosk can also be outsourced to media experts and could expand to handheld devices or to any number of the rapidly evolving technology solutions for information seekers.

Another exciting role for librarians is to participate as an embedded member of physician, nurse, or other clinical interdisciplinary teams to provide point-of-care clinical and patient information services and to review and recommend patient-care resources that caregivers might access virtually. Whether the resulting patient information is written and approved by the organization or are links for providers to appropriate patient-focused websites, the librarian facilitates the clinician's role through instant access to resources for them as well as for their patients. The librarian's embedded role on the healthcare team can be nurtured and nourished through appropriate marketing to targeted professional groups within the organization of its benefits to providers and patients alike.

Government partnerships are another form of strategic collaboration. Aligning the Healthy People 2020 standards with local needs and healthcare priorities builds networks of cross-communication; these can evolve into shared resources, combined skill sets, and common objectives. For example, an organization that has just become "smoke-free" can utilize public resources devoted to this area. This can minimize cost while benefitting patients and employees alike.

As another form of outreach, consumer health librarians can encourage new generations to enter the field by offering mentorships, on-site internships, serving as adjunct professors, or joining chat rooms with library science students. Identifying and communicating consumer health needs can build upon the librarian's professional strengths while opening avenues of discovery for the student. In turn, the students can be invited to lend their expertise by updating websites, developing a library's social media presence, or offering classes on navigating the world of consumer health websites or apps.

Professional affiliations with other local healthcare entities or public libraries can involve co-sponsorship of monthly talks on healthcare topics by specialists, or visits with public librarians or other public agency professionals to learn how their resources complement those of the consumer health library and vice versa. Healthcare Hot Topics programs can be offered either in person or by webcast to library or other patrons, and topical links can be added to consumer health websites or webcasts. In addition, the librarians from public and consumer health libraries can collaborate on collection development to optimize resources at both locations.

Searching online consumer health classes can be taught within the health-care organization and at public libraries, churches, or community or senior centers. Many tools are available to assist, and while consumers increasingly recognize their ability to find information online, they often need assistance in finding reliable information—a task for which the consumer health librarian is ideally suited. In addition, the librarian can "reach out by reaching in" to employees, offering these tips at Lunch and Learn sessions, as articles in employee newsletters, or as part of the institution's health promotion efforts for employees. Completing a pre-teaching survey of interest areas can help the librarian focus specifically on attendees' needs as well as lay a framework for future discussions or classes.

In many healthcare organizations, nursing services are working towards Magnet Certification, a distinction of the very best nursing care, evaluated by a series of standards reflecting nursing empowerment, autonomy, and decision-making (American Nurses Credentialing Center, 2013). The consumer librarian can build partnerships by offering classes for employees on evidence-based practice guidelines, clinical reviews, developing valid searches, and the like, and can demonstrate to surveyors the role the consumer health library offers in regard to health literacy initiatives, patient education resources, and nursing research.

With the focus on evidence-based clinical information, the consumer health librarian can also request membership on the organization's Institutional Review Board, a group that reviews human subject research in the health sciences. The librarian can provide additional focus through highly developed skills to support healthcare research and can also serve as a liaison between the Institutional Review Board and patients by informing patients of study recruitment efforts.

Collaborative relationships can also be forged with public health departments, poison control centers, and similar organizations to distribute timely information to consumers on immunizations, swimming safety, sunburn protection, smoking cessation, and other health promotion efforts. Librarians can provide information from partner agencies on their organization's bulletin boards, in display cases, and in brochure racks in the library.

When institutional funding diminishes, librarians can secure development support either through internal clinical practice grants or externally, through funding from a variety of resources including the National Libraries of Medicine Outreach Grants, Institute of Museum and Library Services, the American Cancer Society, and other disease-specific organizations, including the National Institutes of Health. These monies can be shared with other researchers within the organization on projects that provide mutually beneficial grant dollars for the library along with the clinical areas sponsoring the research.

Conclusion

Collaboration and strategic planning should be a priority in the life of a consumer health librarian, as these not only help sustain the library's mission but support the overall mission and objectives of the organization. Like a garden, tending, watering, nourishing, and harvesting are needed to sustain collaborations over the long term. Time and efforts invested in collaboration and developing strategic partnerships will blossom into an enduring consumer health library offering mature and robust services.

References

American Association of Law Librarians. 2013. "Toolkit Mission Statement." http://www.aallnet.org/sis/pllsis/Toolkit/ToolkitMissionStatement.pdf. Accessed June 1, 2013.

American Nurses Credentialing Center. 2013. ANCC Magnet Recognition Program. http://www.nursecredentialing.org/Magnet.aspx. Accessed June 1, 2013.

Attwood, CA, and Wellik, KE. 2012. "Collaboration, Collegiality, Cooperation: Consumer Health Library and the Role of the American Cancer Society Navigator." *Clinical Journal of Oncology Nursing*, 18(5):487–90.

Drucker, PF. 2008. *The Five Most Important Questions You Will Ever Ask about Your Organization*. San Francisco: Jossey-Bass Publishers.

Internal Revenue Service. 2013. "New Requirements for 501(c)(3) Hospitals under the Affordable Care Act." http://www.irs.gov/Charities-&-Non-Profits/Charitable-Organizations/New-Requirements-for-501%28c%29%283%29-Hospitals-Under-the-Affordable-Care-Act. Accessed September 2, 2013.

Joint Commission. 2013. "About the Joint Commission." http://www.jointcommission.org/about_us/about_the_joint_commission_main.aspx. Accessed June 1, 2013.

Koerner, JE, and Wesley, ML. 2008. "Organizational Culture: The Silent Political Force." *Nursing Administration Quarterly*, 32(1):49–56.

Murray, A. 2010. *The Wall Street Journal Essential Guide to Management*. New York: Harper Business.

National Library of Medicine, National Institutes of Health. 2013. Helping Older Adults Search for Health Information Online Tutorials. http://nihseniorhealth.gov/toolkit/toolkit.html. Accessed June 1, 2013.

Pew Research Center. 2013. Pew Internet and Family Life Project Surveys. http://www.pewinternet.org/. Accessed June 1, 2013.

Stone, J, and Hoffman, GJ. 2010. Congressional Research Services. "Medicare Hospital Readmissions: Issues, Policy Options and PPACA." http://www.ncsl.org/documents/health/Medicare_Hospital_Readmissions_and_PPACA.pdf. Accessed June 1, 2013.

U.S. Department of Health and Human Services, 2013. "Affordable Care Act." Department of Health and Human Services http://www.hhs.gov/opa/affordable-care-act/index.html. Accessed June 1, 2013.

Index

Accountable Care Organization (ACO), 5, 205, 206
Agency for Healthcare Research and Quality (AHRQ), 58, 114, 165
American Academy of Family Physicians, 3, 169; Statement on Patient Education, 3
American Cancer Society, 137, 203, 208
American Diabetes Association, 140
American Heart Association, 138, 139
American Hospital Association, 2, 3
American Library Association, 81, 85, 109, 122, 125, 127
Askanase, D, 192–93
Aurora Healthcare System libraries, 141

Bennett, E, 138
Boston Women's Health Collective, 2
Brigham and Women's Hospital Kessler Health Education Library (Boston), 53
budgeting: books, 44–45; determining needs, 43 (see also needs assessment); equipment, 49; estimating costs, 41–42; facilities and furniture, 49; fiscal year cycles, 42–43; magazines

and newsletters, 45; management, 55; miscellaneous costs, 48; multimedia, 46–47; office supplies, 47–48; Online Public Access Catalog (OPAC), 47; overview, 37–41; pamphlets and brochures, 45; personnel, 50–51 (see also staff); software, 41; training and support, 54

Cave, D, 129
Center for Medicare and Medicaid Services. See Medicare
Centers for Disease Control and Prevention (CDC), 13, 59, 60, 139, 143, 144, 145, 164, 170
Cochrane Collaboration, 69
Collins, SA, 58
Community Health Information Network (Cambridge, MA), 6
Community Health Needs Assessment, 13, 205–6
Consumer and Patient Health Information Section (MLA), 6, 46, 53, 78, 83, 95, 111, 156, 169
Consumer Health Information Consortium (Syracuse, NY), 6

About the Editor

Michele Spatz is currently business projects and intelligence manager for Planetree, a nonprofit healthcare organization devoted to improving both providers' and patients' experience of care. She recently completed work on a grant-funded research project identifying patient-centered care practices among high-performing health systems and academic medical centers outside the Planetree network. In addition to her research responsibilities, Michele executes Planetree's special projects, such as the one noted previously. Michele received her master's degree in library and information science from the University of Illinois, and has a certificate in Lean Six Sigma from Villanova University.

A writer, teacher, and consultant, Michele has over thirty years of experience in the healthcare field. Prior to joining Planetree's international staff in January 2010, Michele helped Mid-Columbia Medical Center, The Dalles, Oregon, implement Planetree's patient-centered care model by organizing, establishing, and directing the Planetree Health Resource Center, building it into a national model for the delivery of patient and consumer health information. Michele led the development of innovative information services to patients and the public for all sectors of the organization and across all continuums of care. She has taught, spoken nationally, and written extensively on reaching patients and consumers with meaningful health information as well as how to design and deliver patient health information programs and services. It is in these roles Michele advocates for patients and consumers alike to be fully engaged partners in their healthcare.

About the Contributors

Carol Ann Attwood, MLS, AHIP, MPH, RN, C, manages the Patient and Health Education Library at Mayo Clinic in Arizona. In her professional career, she has worked as a special education teacher, registered nurse, and medical librarian. Her interests are health literacy, health and wellness, providing resources for patrons with special needs, consumer health collaborations within the community, and librarianship as a second career. She serves on health information services, nursing, and educational groups at her organization, and realizes the importance of collaboration and identifying strategic partnerships and the role that those relationships serve within her consumer health library. She has presented and published in both the nursing and health information profession.

Barbara Bibel is a reference librarian and consumer health information specialist (level II certification from the Medical Library Association) at the Oakland Public Library in California. She has a BA in French from the University of California, Los Angeles, an MA in romance languages from Johns Hopkins University, and an MLS from the University of California, Berkeley. She is the book review editor for the Consumer and Patient Health Information Section of the Medical Library Association and an active reviewer for *Booklist*, *Library Journal*, *American Reference Books Annual*, the Association of Jewish Libraries, and the Jewish Book Council. She trains staff members and the public in searching and evaluating health and medical information.

Jackie Davis, MLIS, has been a librarian for over ten years, working in a military library, a public library, in the world of adult literacy, and now as a consumer health librarian. She has experience as a community organizer and has taken these skills into the library at Sharp Memorial Hospital. Telling others about the health library at her institution is a joy because she believes so strongly in the power of information—especially the power of information embedded in a caring relationship. Among her awards are the 2013 CAPHIS Consumer Health Librarian of the Year award and being named a 2013 Gale/ Cengage Librarian Superhero.

Nicole Dettmar is the education and assessment coordinator for the National Network of Libraries of Medicine, Pacific Northwest Region at the University of Washington Health Sciences Library in Seattle, Washington. She holds a master's of science in information science with a focus in health informatics from the University of North Texas, and a Level II Consumer Health Information Specialization from the Medical Library Association (MLA). Her professional interests include serving as editor of the *Consumer Connections* newsletter for MLA's Consumer and Patient Health Information Section and lead moderator for the weekly #medlibs chat on Twitter.

Nancy Dickenson, MLIS, joined the staff of Stanford Hospital Health Library in 2002. She holds a master's in library and information science from San Jose State University. Active in both the Medical Library Association and the Special Libraries Association, Nancy served on the International Federation of Libraries Association standing committee on Information Literacy and is a past chair of SLA's Biomedical and Life Sciences Division.

Mary Grace Flaherty is currently an assistant professor at the School of Information and Library Science at the University of North Carolina at Chapel Hill. She received her PhD as an IMLS Fellow at Syracuse University's iSchool and her MLS from the University of Maryland. She received her MS in applied behavioral science from Johns Hopkins University. Mary Grace has over twenty years of experience working in a variety of positions in library settings, including academic, medical research, and as a director of a public library. Her research interests include consumer health information, health literacy, and libraries.

Carmen Huddleston, MLIS, is a librarian with Stanford Hospital Health Library, based in the hospital branch. Before she came to Stanford in 2007, Carmen worked as a research associate with a pharmaceutical database company. She received her master's in library and information science from San Jose State University. Carmen is the current chair for the Northern California and Nevada Medical Librarians Group.

Jean Johnson, MLIS, came to Stanford Hospital Health Library as a volunteer in 2008. She became a staff librarian in 2011. Prior to joining the staff, Jean has been a librarian for more than twenty years with positions at public and special libraries in New York and California. Jean received her master's in library and information science from the University of Illinois at Urbana-Champaign.

Michelle A. Kraft is the senior medical librarian at the Cleveland Clinic Alumni Library. She is the author of *The Krafty Librarian*, a blog for medical librarians, writing primarily about technology, medical libraries, and librarianship. Michelle can also be found tweeting as @krafty on medical library issues and is a regular participant of the #medlibs Twitter chat group. Among her traditional library duties she is currently working with the Cleveland Clinic Education Institute to test the use of Google+ as an internal institutional networking and discussion site to foster a more efficient group work environment and to lessen the silo effect common in large institutions.

Michelle has authored several articles and spoken often on the use of technology within medical libraries and on the evolving medical library user. She has been a panelist and moderator for the Medical Informatics Section and Educational Media & Technologies Section popular *Top Technology Trends* program. She has also been a panelist on two Medical Library Association Educational Webcasts on the use of technology and medical libraries. Michelle received her MLS from the University of Missouri–Columbia and is member of the Academy of Health Information Professionals, Medical Library Association, Midwest Medical Library Association, and the Ohio Health Sciences Library Association.

Gillian Kumagai, MLIS, AHIP, has worked at Stanford Hospital Health Library since 2004 and is the librarian in the Stanford Cancer Center branch. She is actively involved in the Consumer and Patient Health Information Section of the Medical Library Association, the Division of Biomedical and Life Sciences of the Special Libraries Association, along with other library-related organizations. Gillian received her master's in library and information science from San Jose State University.

Erica Lake joined the Spencer S. Eccles Health Sciences Library in 2011 as associate librarian, and is associate director of the Hope Fox Eccles Health

Library, a consumer health library located in University Hospital. In this role, Erica ensures that patients, their families, and the general community have access to the services and resources they need to make informed choices about their healthcare.

Erica earned her MLS from Indiana University, and worked in academic, public, and special libraries before entering the field of hospital librarianship in 1999. She was a senior medical librarian at Intermountain Healthcare for eleven years, where she worked to increase clinical access to evidence-based information and played a leadership role in coordinating corporate-wide availability of electronic biomedical resources. In 2004, she received the Barbara McDowell Award for Excellence in Hospital Librarianship from the Mid-continental Chapter of the Medical Library Association.

Edgar López, MSLS, has been a librarian at Stanford Hospital Health Library since 2011. Previously, he was a graduate library assistant for the University Archives and the music library at the University of North Texas. In addition, he was also a teaching assistant for both the College of Information and the Department of Kinesiology, Health Promotion, and Recreation at the University of North Texas. Edgar received his master of science degree in library science from the University of North Texas, where he has a doctoral degree in process.

Cara Marcus, MSLIS, AHIP, is director of library services for Brigham and Women's Faulkner Hospital. She oversees operations of the Medical Library and Patient/Family Resource Center and is resources chair for the Patient/Family Education Committee. Cara was president of the Massachusetts Health Sciences Library Network during 2013/2014 and is chair of the Medical Library Association committee that publishes *Managing a Consumer Health Information Service*. She writes reviews of consumer health books for MLA *Consumer Connections* and *Journal of Consumer Health on the Internet* and is the author of *Images of America: Faulkner Hospital* (2010).

Donna J. McCloskey has been the manager of library services at Novant Health Huntersville Medical Center in Huntersville, North Carolina, since the hospital's opening in 2004. Donna earned her bachelor of arts in English from California State University, Chico, and master of library and information science from the University of South Carolina. She holds a Level II designation in the Medical Library Association's Consumer Health Information Specialization and is a member of the Academy of Health Information Professionals. Donna was the recipient of the MLA, Hospital Libraries Section, Catch a Rising Star award in 2007. She is the co-editor of the Patchwork column in the *Journal of Hospital Librarianship* and a frequent contributor of articles and reviews for that journal, the *Journal of the Medical Library Association*, and other medical library publications.

Emma O'Hagan is a medical librarian at the University of Western Michigan School of Medicine. Previously, Emma was a reference librarian at the Lister Hill Library of the Health Sciences at the University of Alabama at Birmingham (UAB) where she also worked at the Kirklin Clinic Patient Resource Library located in UAB's outpatient clinic. At the clinic library, she helped patients identify resources to help them better understand their healthcare. Emma has taught mobile technology classes and workshops for the WMed and UAB communities, and develops and maintains guides for using mobile medical resources.

Gabe Rios is the deputy director of the Lister Hill Library of the Health Sciences at the University of Alabama at Birmingham. Gabe has worked with emerging technologies since the late 1990s. He has taught technology-related classes at regional and national meetings over the past ten years. Gabe has also served as a member of national and local technology groups such as the MLA Technology Advisory Committee, Alabama Social Media Association, and the Internet Professional Society of Alabama. Gabe is a devoted user of technology and has a keen interest in technology trends and their impact on librarianship.

Jean Shipman is director, Spencer S. Eccles Health Sciences Library and the MidContinental Region and National Training Center of the National Network of Libraries of Medicine at the University of Utah. She served as president of the Medical Library Association for 2006–2007 and promoted health literacy as her primary presidential initiative. Jean graduated from CWRU and Gettysburg College. She has worked in academic health sciences libraries (Johns Hopkins University, University of Washington, VCU), a hospital library (Greater Baltimore Medical Center), and with the Southeastern/Atlantic NN/LM at the University of Maryland, Baltimore. Her professional interests include health literacy, library administration, scholarly communications, and innovation and LEAN principles.

Linda Stahl, coordinator of the Planetree Health Resource Center, in The Dalles, Oregon, has provided consumer health information to patients at Mid-Columbia Medical Center (MCMC) and individuals in her community for the past twenty-one years. Mid-Columbia Medical Center is a Designated Planetree Hospital, meaning it meets the standards for the highest quality patient-centered care. A large component of the patient-centered model is patient access to information. Her role as coordinator of the Planetree Health Resource Center includes managing the consumer health collection of over three thousand titles for the public, and meeting MCMC patients' information needs through novel services such as providing patient information packets through patient rounds and coordinating various community outreach projects, including co-chair of the Go Red for Women's Heart Health community education event each February. She has published articles in the *Journal of Hospital Librarianship* and *Journal of Consumer Health on the Internet* on writing and searching for reliable health information in plain language.

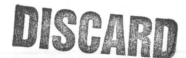